MW00562847

Partner Workouts

Training Together for Better Results

Krista Popowych

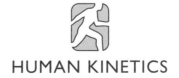

HUMAN KINETICS

Library of Congress Cataloging-in-Publication Data

Names: Popowych, Krista, 1970- author.
Title: Partner workouts: training together for better results / Krista
 Popowych.
Description: Champaign, IL : Human Kinetics, [2022] | Includes
 bibliographical references.
Identifiers: LCCN 2021022641 (print) | LCCN 2021022642 (ebook) | ISBN
 9781718200401 (paperback) | ISBN 9781718200418 (epub) | ISBN
 9781718200425 (pdf)
Subjects: LCSH: Exercise for couples. | Physical fitness.
Classification: LCC GV481 .P585 2022 (print) | LCC GV481 (ebook) | DDC
 613.7--dc23
LC record available at https://lccn.loc.gov/2021022641
LC ebook record available at https://lccn.loc.gov/2021022642

ISBN: 978-1-7182-0040-1 (print)

Senior Acquisitions Editor: Michelle Earle; **Developmental Editor:** Amy Stahl; **Copyeditor:** Lisa Himes; **Proofreader:** Erin Cler; **Senior Graphic Designer:** Nancy Rasmus; **Cover Designer:** Keri Evans; **Cover Design Specialist:** Susan Rothermel Allen; **Photograph (cover):** Emir Memedovski / Getty Images; **Photographs (interior):** Rick Etkin Productions/© Human Kinetics; **Photo Production Specialist:** Amy M. Rose; **Photo Production Manager:** Jason Allen; **Senior Art Manager:** Kelly Hendren; **Illustrations:** © Human Kinetics; **Printer:** Versa Press

We thank Richmond Olympic Oval in Richmond, British Columbia, Canada, for assistance in providing the location for the photo shoot for this book.

Human Kinetics books are available at special discounts for bulk purchase. Special editions or book excerpts can also be created to specification. For details, contact the Special Sales Manager at Human Kinetics.

Printed in the United States of America   10   9   8   7   6   5   4   3   2   1

The paper in this book is certified under a sustainable forestry program.

Human Kinetics	*United States and International*	*Canada*
1607 N. Market Street	Website: **US.HumanKinetics.com**	Website: **Canada.HumanKinetics.com**
Champaign, IL 61820	Email: info@hkusa.com	Email: info@hkcanada.com
USA	Phone: 1-800-747-4457	

E8176

Tell us what you think!
Human Kinetics would love to hear what we
can do to improve the customer experience.
Use this QR code to take our brief survey.

This book is dedicated to Mom and Dad,
Teresa, Jennifer, Lou, Jared, and Layla.
You are my everything.

CONTENTS

PART I   GET SET

PART II   PARTNER EXERCISES

PART III SAMPLE WORKOUTS

EXERCISE FINDER

Exercise	Challenge level	Bodyweight training	Resistance band	Medicine ball	Cardio focused	Page number
CHAPTER 5: BODYWEIGHT EXERCISES						
Back Extension	Easy	x				73
Bicycle Crunch	Moderate	x				69
Crab and Reach	Moderate	x				60
Curl-Up and Give Me 10	Moderate	x				68
Down Dog Crawl	Moderate	x				58
Front Squat Hold	Easy	x				50
Get-Ups	Moderate	x				48
Handstand	Hard	x				66
Kneeling Push-Up With Rotation	Easy	x				63
Pistol Squat	Hard	x				49
Plank and Push-Up	Hard	x				64
Plank and Row	Hard	x				55
Reverse Tabletop and Triceps Dip	Hard	x				53
Snowboarder	Hard	x			x	61
Squat and Glute Lift	Hard	x				51
Straight-Leg Lift	Moderate	x				67
Surfer Pop-Up	Hard	x			x	62
Tabletop and Jumping Jack	Hard	x			x	52
Up-and-Over Abs	Hard	x				72
V-Sit Circle	Moderate	x				71
Walk Out and Clap	Moderate	x				57
Wheelbarrow Push-Up and Squat	Hard	x				56

(continued)

Exercise	Challenge level	Bodyweight training	Resistance band	Medicine ball	Cardio focused	Page number
CHAPTER 6: PARTNER-RESISTED EXERCISES						
Back-to-Back Walkout	Hard	x				77
Glute Bridge Bicycle	Hard	x				84
Glute Bridge Lift	Hard	x				83
Leg Press	Hard	x				80
Lunge and Press	Moderate	x				79
Pushover Press	Easy	x				78
Resisted Front and Side Raise	Easy	x				85
Resisted Hamstring Curl	Easy	x				82
Resisted Oblique Curl	Easy	x				91
Resisted Push-Up	Easy	x				87
Resisted Tabletop	Easy	x				86
Rotating Side Planks	Moderate	x				90
Side Plank Hold	Moderate	x				88
Wall Sit	Hard	x				76
CHAPTER 7: SMALL-EQUIPMENT EXERCISES						
Ball Slam	Moderate			x		99
Biceps Curl and Side Lunge	Moderate		x			117
Boxing Jabs	Easy		x			122
Chest Press	Easy		x			116
Curl-Up and Pass	Moderate			x		102
Football Run	Moderate		x		x	107
Forward and Backward Lunge and Pass	Moderate			x		96
Front Press and Leap	Moderate		x		x	111
High Row With Wide Squat	Easy		x			119
Lateral Lunge and Toss	Moderate			x		97
Long Jump	Moderate		x		x	112
Lunge and Rotation	Moderate		x			114

Exercise	Challenge level	Bodyweight training	Resistance band	Medicine ball	Cardio focused	Page number
Oblique Band Curl	Moderate		x			127
Parachute Band Run	Hard		x			110
Rock and Curl	Moderate		x			126
Row and Hop Back	Moderate		x		x	113
Seated Pass With Rotation	Moderate			x		104
Side Shuffle	Moderate		x		x	108
Sit and Pass	Moderate			x		103
Skier	Hard		x		x	106
Squat to Side Pass	Moderate			x		94
Tap-Down Abs	Moderate		x			124
Triceps Kickback	Easy		x			123
Trunk Rotation	Easy		x			120
Uneven Push-Up and Roll	Moderate			x		100
Woodchopper	Moderate			x		95
CHAPTER 8: CARDIO AND HIIT EXERCISES						
Burpee Jumps	Hard	x			x	134
Curl-Up and Jumping Jack	Hard	x			x	145
Donkey Kick	Hard	x			X	138
Follow the Leader	Easy	x			x	130
High-Knees Run	Moderate	x			x	131
Leapfrog	Moderate	x			x	133
Long Jump and High Jump	Hard	x			x	139
Narrow Push-Up and Hop Over	Hard	x			x	144
Plank Leap	Hard	x			x	137
Resisted Run	Hard	x			x	132
Rotating Squat Jump	Hard	x			x	141
Squat Jump to High 10	Hard	x			x	140
Walkout Ankle Taps	Moderate	x			x	142
Wide Plank and Agility Footwork	Hard	x			x	136

(continued)

Exercise	Challenge level	Bodyweight training	Resistance band	Medicine ball	Cardio focused	Page number
CHAPTER 9: PARTNER SOLO EXERCISES						
Burpee	Hard	x			x	150
Fast Run–Squat	Hard	x			x	151
Front and Back Lunge	Moderate	x				153
Half-Arc Press	Moderate	x				156
Jumping Jack	Easy	x			x	148
Low Jack	Moderate	x			x	149
Mountain Climber	Moderate	x			x	151
Offset Push-Up	Hard	x				155
Out–In Squat Walk	Moderate	x				152
Plank With Arm Extended	Hard	x				154
Pull-Through Abs	Hard	x				155
Running on the Spot	Easy	x			x	149
Side Lunge With Reach	Moderate	x				153
Squat, Touch, Lift	Easy	x				152
T-Back Pulls	Easy	x				154
CHAPTER 10: FLEXIBILITY TRAINING EXERCISES						
Back Stretch	Easy	x				159
Calf and Hip Flexor Stretch	Easy	x				160
Chest Stretch	Easy	x				158
Glute Stretch	Easy	x				160
Hamstring and Upper Back Stretch	Easy	x				159
Quadriceps Stretch	Easy	x				158

PREFACE

The use of partner workouts is an interactive and engaging training strategy to inspire you to get stronger and more fit while exercising with a friend or workout partner. This shared style of exercise puts a creative spin on working out beyond traditional training methods. What makes partner workouts unique is that each person becomes an active part of the exercise program. Whether it's passing a medicine ball during an abdominal exercise, leaping over each other's legs in a cardio drill, or creating resistance by pressing against each other's feet in a bridge exercise, each person plays an important role in the workout. Each participant becomes the primary exercise tool in the fitness equipment toolbox.

Partner Workouts provides a wide range of exercise suggestions and workout plans that are creative, inspiring, and mutually beneficial to each participant. The majority of the exercises are based on bodyweight training, with no equipment required. Other exercise combinations use commonly available and easily accessible equipment such as resistance bands or medicine balls. These tools enhance the training and keep partners connected. The workouts can also be performed almost anywhere. Whether at home, in a studio, or outdoors, all that is required is a bit of space and a willing partner. The versatility of partner training program design makes the workouts adaptable and scalable.

Within this book, you will learn creative and effective ways to put together interesting partner exercises and routines. These combinations will then become the basis of various workout regimes. Some exercises are more cardio-based, whereas others are more equipment-based. Certain exercises may be body-part specific or may include a combination of upper body, lower body, and core exercises. In some formats, one partner may be engaged in a particular fitness component, while the other person is doing something totally different. This allows and encourages partners with different fitness skills and abilities to feel successful during the workout. The beauty of the exercises in *Partner Workouts* is that you can create your own exercise program or follow one of the many preplanned workouts found in part III that are designed with various goals in mind.

Partner Workouts will provide you with all the necessary programming and exercise information to feel successful. Various formats will be discussed, including simultaneous partner exercise, modality workouts, or partner-resisted exercise. With goal setting, exercise descriptions, recommended equipment, step-by-step partner positioning, movement tips, how-to instructions, progression and regression suggestions for all levels, and specific exercise photos, you can successfully perform each of the exercises and become inspired to create your own combinations or workouts.

ACKNOWLEDGMENTS

Like so many things in our lives, individual success is truly not individual. Rather, success is made possible through the support, encouragement, love, and kindness of those around us who help fuel our accomplishments. I am incredibly grateful to so many who have been on this amazing journey with me.

Thank you to all my family and friends. To my mom and dad, Jerry and Millie Popowych, and my sisters, Teresa Ross and Jennifer Popowych: I love you. Because of our incredible bond and because of each of you, anything is possible. To my husband, Lou Maznik, who has been by my side every step of the way with unconditional love and support: You vowed to stand by me, and you have never wavered. To my amazing children, Jared Maznik and Layla Maznik: You truly are my everything: my light, my love, and my whole being.

It takes a village. To my dream team, my sisters: I thank you. Words can't describe how grateful and appreciative I am of your incredible talents and unwavering support. Thank you to Davey Ross, Christopher Ross, Jared Maznik, Layla Maznik, Kenzie McMaster, Gabrielle Rossignol, and Amanda Lau for gracing each of the pages with your talents and love. To my behind-the-scenes supporters, Ashton McMaster, Stu McMaster, and David Ross: I thank you.

To my dear friends, Natalie Way, Chantal Laurin, Jacquie Stebbings, Johanna Oosthuizen, and Cristin Corneille: You are my rocks. You each make my life richer and more fun. Thank you for your kindness and support.

I would not be where I am today had I not walked through the doors of The Fitness Group so many years ago and met incredible leaders and visionaries like Barbara Crompton and Julie Milner. You taught me so much and always encouraged me. A special thank you to my fitness colleagues and champions, Paco Gonzáles, Suzette O'Byrne, and Amanda Vogel.

Thank you to my dedicated editors at Human Kinetics, Michelle Earle and Amy Stahl, for asking me to do this project and being there every step of the way. You are so talented, patient, and kind.

Lastly, I would like to thank every student I have ever taught and every teacher, colleague, and mentor whom I have learned from and been inspired by. Through you, I have been able to share my passion for fitness and education, pursue my goals, inspire others, and live my best life.

INTRODUCTION

As a child, I have fond memories of playing with my dad. Lying on the floor, he would lift me and my sisters up onto his feet for make-believe airplane rides, or we would hop on his back for piggyback rides around the living room floor. I remember skipping rope with my mom while reciting jump rope rhymes. Add in tug-of-war, wheelbarrow, and three-legged races at sports days, and these could be considered my earliest introduction to partner workouts—without knowing that these activities might be considered exercise. I also grew up in an era in which playing outside from sunrise to sunset was the norm for most kids, and suggesting to our parents that we might be bored was an automatic invitation to be given something unexciting to do, like a chore. With that in mind, exercise wasn't something separate from work or play; being active was how we lived our lives.

My passion for fitness continued to grow as I got older. My sisters and I often gravitated to whatever each other did, and this included playing basketball, volleyball, and other sports, or activities like chopping wood or challenging our cousins to a log rolling contest at the cabin. I loved being active.

By the time I was in my early twenties, the aerobics craze hit, and I was introduced to the world of group fitness. Turning my passion for movement into a career was a decision I have never regretted. I studied human kinetics, said "yes" to any fitness-related opportunity, gained as much exercise and presenting experience as I could, and was fortunate to be mentored throughout my career by talented and giving industry leaders.

I also deeply believe in the power of staying active. Choosing to exercise and move your body every day, like brushing your teeth, is a necessity that brings positive and lifelong benefits. But that doesn't mean it has to be intimidating or boring. It should make you feel better and not worse, be engaging and worth heading out the door for, and dare I say, fun. Its benefits, even on a difficult day, far outweigh its challenges.

Whether I am teaching a group exercise class, training, or presenting fitness-based curriculum across the globe, my goal has always been to inspire others through movement and education. And to do so in a way that is real and applies to everyday life—not too fancy or complicated.

"Simplicity is the ultimate sophistication" in the words of Leonardo DaVinci. Fitness is a lifelong journey, but it's not always easy. Sometimes we fall off the path, and that's okay. We just have to get back up and keep trying until we find something that works.

I want to inspire you, my children, my family, and my friends with the power of exercise, and to help change our collective mindset and subsequent dialogue from "I have to work out" to "I get to work out." My hope is that you enjoy and are motivated by the partner exercises in this book. They are meant to be fun and effective and keep you and your workout buddy inspired to enjoy each part of your individual fitness journey, together.

Partner Workouts is separated into three main sections. Part I discusses the many benefits of training with a partner and reviews key fitness components, including cardiovascular, strength, and flexibility training. It continues to explain the foundations of training, discusses how to make partner workouts successful with partner roles and goals as well as proper space and equipment tips. Part II explores the how-tos and includes a library of exercise ideas for bodyweight training, partner-resisted, small-equipment, cardio and HIIT, solo exercises, and flexibility training. Part III provides samples of different training workouts to guide you and your partner, based on your workout goals, needs, and interests. Appendix A offers tips and suggestions specific to personal trainers and how they can incorporate partner workouts into their business offerings. Appendix B includes a SWEAT goal setting sheet for yourself or to complete with your partner.

Let's begin your journey into *Partner Workouts*!

PART I

GET SET

Jumping in with two feet, or in this case four feet, is a stepping-stone on an exciting path of exercising together. One of the biggest benefits of partner workouts is the camaraderie that naturally occurs. Whether it is working toward a common goal, being there for each other, or any of the mind–body–spirit benefits, it is about connecting physically in more ways than one. A firm foundation of basic fitness knowledge further solidifies a successful partnership, and building on this know-how is a peripheral benefit of preparation. As you get started, it is important to carve out a personal workout space, regardless of size, and invest in some small equipment pieces for you and your partner. Lastly, with any workout plan, everyone needs a role. Defining how to best fit that role and how to maximize your time together by setting goals will lead to greater partner workout success and more enjoyment.

CHAPTER 1

Benefits of Partner Workouts

Currently, we have never been more connected via social networking and virtual communities, yet we have also become physically disconnected. Whether by choice or due to global circumstance, face-to-face contact is not always an everyday reality. However, if we reminisce about our favorite personal and memorable moments, chances are we didn't experience those events alone. Spending time with someone else, regardless of what it is, increases our enjoyment factor. That's why partner workouts are popular. Working out with a friend or colleague creates a different exercise environment and energy. Training together also facilitates camaraderie and teamwork. It inspires goal setting and encourages commitment. But most importantly, it makes working out more interesting, interactive, and fun.

Exercise Adherence

Imagine typical new or returning exercisers. Walking into a gym for the first time, they often feel intimidated. They have ventured into a new environment filled with unfamiliar pieces of fitness equipment populated by fitness buffs plugged into headphones or sporting Lycra. In addition to not knowing where or how to get started, also noticeable is the interactions between members. Conversation is limited, and typically only one person can use a piece of cardio or strength equipment at a time. Certainly, this is not the case in all facilities, but it can be daunting for the new person, and an environment perhaps better suited to those who like to exercise alone.

However, training solo isn't for everyone. In contrast, peek into a group fitness class or a small-group training session and the scene is markedly different. Exercisers appear engaged, and a collective focus on achieving a group goal creates a unique experience, even if it is simply getting through the session or class together. A motivated instructor leads the charge, and training partners chat with each other while working out. Friends gather after the session and there are noticeably more smiles. Increased positive interactions, albeit in the novel environment of a gym or while doing something challenging, seem to boost the enjoyment factor.

If interactions with another like-minded individual can bring greater enjoyment to things that we must do, like staying active and eating well, partner workouts is a great way to program for success. Often cited in exercise adherence and physical activity goal-setting research, social interactions while working out with someone and receiving ongoing support from family and friends are strong predictors of exercise adherence. The workout buddy plan guides and helps people stick to their goals.

Occasionally, we all need an extra push to get our workouts done, and committing to someone else helps. There is also the guilt. Our conscience gets the best of us if we cancel. Plus, we don't want the fallout associated with ghosting a friend if we bail on them or forget to show up. A workout buddy significantly increases adherence and keeps us bound to what we say we will do. Half the battle of a successful workout regime is won by simply showing up.

Time Saver

Not having enough time or failing to set aside time to exercise is high on the list of excuses for not working out. In fact, time, or the perceived lack thereof, still remains the number one reason for skipping regular exercise, irrespective of the wasted hours that society spends on their smartphones or streaming the latest Netflix docuseries. But time is not the only excuse. Other factors affecting exercise participation include being unsure of what to do, feeling physically uncomfortable, a real or perceived fear of getting injured, boredom, lack of equipment, not wanting to be in a gym environment, and negative past experiences associated with exercise. By training with a partner, many of these shared challenges can be better managed and perhaps even eliminated. Partner workouts provide options such as shorter routines, less or no equipment, and the possibility of exercising together in the comfort and privacy of your own home.

Partner workouts do not require equipment. In several of the exercises, the partner becomes the actual resistance. Whether it is performing a move simultaneously to increase effort, such as linking arms together while squatting back-to-back, or adding resistance to a push-up by placing your hands on your partner's back, the resistance is generated through the movement or partner. No equipment is needed. Bodyweight training continues to be popular because it is simple and effective and can streamline workout time by eliminating equipment needs.

If equipment is used in partner workouts, it can easily be shared. Requiring two of everything is no longer necessary. For example, when using a resistance band, one partner can be the anchor by holding one end of the band, and the other partner can do the exercise; then the roles are switched. One medicine ball can be used in a catch–release drill. A mat can be used to cushion a curl-up while the other partner is upright and performing a lunge. With experience and regular training, partners may even design new or unique partner exercises using their own equipment.

With time being our modern-day currency, minutes also matter. Performing challenging partner exercises allows more to be done in less time because, when an exercise is physically taxing, fewer reps are required. In addition, working out together means the time between sets is well used. If one partner is doing an exercise, the other can be assisting or motivating them, or using the time to actively recover between sets.

Partner workouts can be done almost anywhere, anytime. Any open studio or gym space that comfortably fits two people can accommodate a workout. The same applies to at-home training. Clear a room, work out in a garage, or hit an outdoor court or park. The perks of this style of training are that it is incredibly versatile, scalable to all fitness enthusiasts, and can be done at various locations.

Physical Benefits

Another benefit beyond the interesting exercises and the commitment perks of partner workouts is the physiological and psychological benefits. Physiologically, all components of a well-designed exercise program should be addressed. Partner workouts include the three fitness components that are the training anchors of any exercise plan or sports-performance training regime: cardiovascular fitness, muscular fitness, and flexibility training (see figure 1.1). Personal and physical goals will dictate what percentage of training time is spent in each anchor. For example, a marathon runner will spend more of her time training her cardiorespiratory system. Even though improving the aerobic system is key, long distance runners also need to be strong and flexible. They must still commit the time, albeit less, to strength and flexibility training. In this scenario, strength training builds a better foundation and improves running stride, and flexibility training enhances muscular performance and reduces running-related injuries. If one of the anchors is missing, regardless of the chosen activity, an exercise program becomes unbalanced and less effective. The marathoner may not be able to run to his optimal potential if he ignores one of the components.

We often interchange the terms *physical activity* and *exercise*. Physical activity is all-encompassing. When we move our bodies in a way that takes effort and expends energy in the form of calorie burning, we are physically active. Walking the dog, cleaning the house, and raking leaves are all examples of physical activities. Exercise is one of the categories found under the umbrella of physical activity. Exercise is defined as focused physical effort having a specific goal to improve overall fitness and health (Magal and Scheinowitz 2018). Exercise is usually planned, whereas physical activity involves daily task-oriented events.

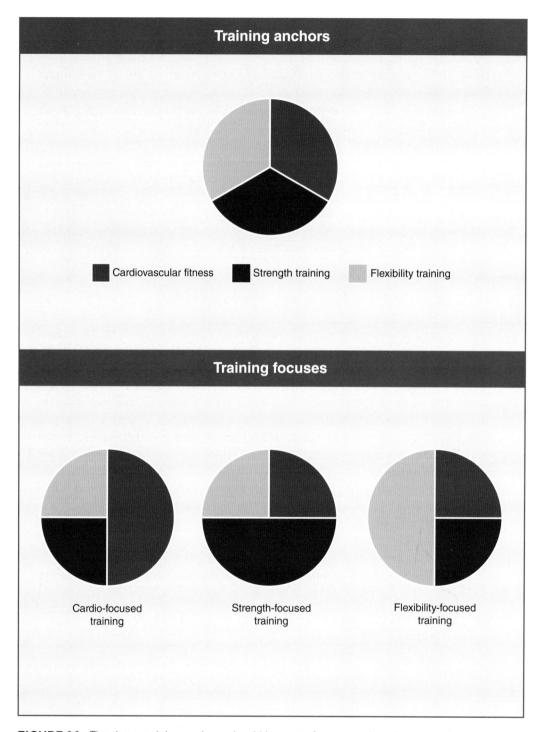

FIGURE 1.1 The three training anchors should be part of any exercise plan or sports-performance training regime. The training focus—cardio, strength, or flexibility—will determine the percentage of each anchor in an individual's workout.

Recently, there has been a greater push toward increasing an individual's amount of nonexercise activity thermogenesis (NEAT), which is the amount of energy expended for all activities executed outside of sleeping, eating, or exercising (Kravitz 2006). Examples of NEAT are simple tasks such as getting out of your office chair more often, walking during your lunch break, and parking your car farther away from your desired location. Even that annoying nervous fidgeting that your partner does is included. Simply stated, it is movement outside of structured exercise or activities. The goal is to move more throughout the day and increase caloric expenditure associated with NEAT.

There are many examples that highlight how inactive people have become. Years ago, sitting idly when there was always work to be done was not a common practice, but we are now faced with an epidemic of chronic sitters. A day in the life of most nonlaboring North Americans typically follows a standard pattern: wake up, dress, sit and eat breakfast, sit in our cars or in transit to commute to our jobs. At work, whether at home or on-site, continue to sit at lunch, coffee breaks, and in meetings. Commute home. Sit at dinner. This is followed by more hours of stationary activities such as watching TV or Internet surfing, and then it's off to bed. In this scenario, less than one hour of a 16-hour waking cycle is spent in movement-related activities.

If the "sitting disease" is detrimental to health, movement is the medicine. The need for a well-structured exercise plan like partner workouts encourages less inactivity and more movement, with a goal to increase all nonstructured fitness as well. If we feel fit and strong, we are more likely to be active throughout the day. Exercise is by far the best thing we can do for ourselves and those around us.

In addition to many of the nonexercise-related benefits of partner workouts, there are also many physical benefits. To get started, let's look at the three anchors of exercise programming and how they can be applied to partner workouts.

Cardiovascular Fitness

Cardiovascular fitness, sometimes referred to as cardiorespiratory endurance, is the ability of the circulatory and respiratory system to supply oxygen during sustained physical activity (Magal and Scheinowitz 2018). Performing large-muscle, repetitive, moderate- to high-intensity exercise for extended periods of time is an example of cardiovascular fitness. The cardiorespiratory system is primarily composed of the heart, lungs, and blood vessels (arteries, capillaries, veins). The heart is a muscular pump that circulates the oxygen and nutrient-rich blood to all the tissues and organs of the body via blood vessels and pumps deoxygenated blood to the lungs. The respiratory system ensures every cell in the body is constantly receiving oxygen and getting rid of carbon dioxide via the lungs and airways.

A 20-minute jog, sprinting laps around a track, or swimming laps in a pool are all examples of cardiovascular exercise. A disease-free cardiovascular system that can effectively respond to the demands of daily living, physical activity, and exercise is crucial to staying healthy (Riebe 2015). But not all cardio exercise is the same. Some low-intensity, long-duration exercises raise heart and breathing rates only slightly. Other exercises are moderate in both intensity and duration, while still others can be extremely demanding with high intensities that cause breathing and heart rates to spike. Muscles require higher oxygen levels when exercise is intense. The by-product of breathing faster is a higher heart rate and the need to remove carbon dioxide faster (McCall 2019). Heart rate, like rating of perceived exertion, is a good measure of intensity.

All exercise requires energy produced from the chemical breakdown of ATP (adenosine triphosphate) at the cellular level. Immediately when we start to exercise, the body begins to resynthesize ATP from one of three energy pathways. These three pathways are (1) immediate sources that use stored energy in the form of creatine phosphate (ATP-CP energy system); (2) glycolysis and glycogenolysis, which use blood glucose and stored muscle glycogen (anaerobic energy system); and (3) oxidative (aerobic energy) system, which uses carbohydrates, fat, and protein metabolism (Potteiger 2018). The energy produced during exercise must match utilization during exercise, or the intensity must be reduced or stopped. For example, exercising as hard as possible for two minutes increases the formation of lactic acid and subsequent fatigue, and the lactic acid buildup forces an athlete to slow down or stop (Potteiger 2018).

A style of cardio training included in partner workouts is HIIT training. HIIT (high-intensity interval training) is an enhanced form of interval training that alternates extremely hard bouts of work with recovery periods. Going full out during true HIIT relies on your anaerobic pathways to produce the immediate energy needed. The energy required to fuel the interval is limited, so the amount of time an individual can sustain the intense efforts is short. Proper recovery time is necessary in order to repeat the work sets at a similar intensity. The harder the work set, the longer the recovery time needed. HIIT is not a new form of exercise; the first recorded trainings were noted in the early 1900s with Olympic runners in Finland using a more systematic approach (Magness 2016). Fitness professionals and enthusiasts like the boost-and-recovery format for efficient workouts.

There are many other benefits to HIIT. Most significant is an increase in resting metabolic rate after a workout due to an increase in excess postexercise oxygen consumption (EPOC). After an exercise session, oxygen consumption, and consequently caloric expenditure, remains elevated as the working muscle cells restore physiological and metabolic factors in the cell to preexercise levels. This translates into higher and longer calorie burning after exercise has stopped (Kravitz 2014). Other benefits include improvement in $\dot{V}O_2$max, better athletic performance of well-trained athletes, increased fat burning and lower insulin levels, improved skeletal-muscle fat oxidation, and improved glucose tolerance. HIIT training improves the health of recreational exercisers and enhances the fitness goals of athletes (Zuhl and Kravitz 2012). Plus in a time-crunched society, HIIT provides many of the benefits of continuous-endurance training but in fewer workouts (Daussin et al. 2008).

Finding enough time to exercise is an ongoing issue, so getting more done in less time is ideal. The format of interval training, whether it's scientific-designed HIIT or a modified version, complements partner workouts well. The back-and-forth play from intensity to recovery provides opportunities for active rest between the work sets. Chapter 8 includes a variety of cardio-based partner interval sets and a breakdown of various HIIT formats to experience, including Tabatas, progressive intervals, and more.

Muscular Fitness

In addition to cardiovascular training, muscular fitness includes both muscular strength and muscular endurance training. Partner workouts balance the benefits of both. Being strong is important for everyday tasks such as lifting heavy objects and is improved through muscular strength training. Muscular strength is defined as the force the muscle can generate in one maximal effort (Boldt 2018). Lifting a heavy carry-on bag from the ground up to the overhead compartment in a plane is an example of muscular strength. Muscular endurance is defined as the ability of the muscle to generate repeated contractions or to sustain a contraction (Boldt 2018). Being able to hold a heavy object for a long time, such as carrying bags of groceries home from the supermarket, requires muscular endurance.

Flexibility Training

The third important component of exercise programming is flexibility training. Flexibility is defined as the range of motion (ROM) available around the joint and is joint specific (Thompson 2008). Movement around a healthy joint should be confined to the joint's functional range of motion. The cartilage, ligaments, tendons, muscle fascia, and fascia sheath make up some of the connective tissues of the joint and have very characteristic functions. In addition, there are many factors that influence and affect flexibility such as age, the elasticity of ligaments and tendons, and even gender. Women are more flexible than men across most ages (Valdivia et al. 2009). Developing a stretching program with a partner is an ideal way to incorporate flexibility goals that complement various activities and sports. Stretching with a partner can range from holding basic static poses to more advanced training using proprio-neuromuscular facilitation (PNF) or active-isolated types of stretching.

Psychological Benefits

Partner workouts promote cognitive and communication skills, and allow you to practice being present in the training processes. Working together cooperatively and building a strong foundation is the key to success to any great partnership. Psychologically, spending time and exercising with a partner, whether a friend, family member, or workout buddy, brings positive social interaction opportunities. Research has shown that creating connections through social bonds is one of the most important factors in life satisfaction (Setton et al. 2021; Bergland 2016). Simply put, being with people makes us happier. An even more beneficial long-term reward is that the happier we are, the more likely we are to continue taking care of ourselves, thus gravitating toward additional healthier outlets and positive lifestyle choices beyond exercise.

Exercise produces natural endorphins, the feel-good hormones that heighten our feelings of happiness. It also produces other benefits like appetite suppression and immune-system enhancements. Experiencing a postworkout "runner's high" keeps regular fitness enthusiasts coming back, and is most likely why they enjoy working out.

If we ask our unmotivated or workout-reluctant friends if exercise is fun, some would likely answer with an emphatic no. Understandable. Exercise is very challenging when we are out of shape. It is intimidating when we don't know what to do. It can also be embarrassing when we feel lost or we don't look like or self-identify with the rest of the gym community. However, partner workouts can mitigate many of these fears. Getting into a regular workout routine with a friend who is also a nonexerciser is a great stepping-stone to making exercise a lifelong habit. Together you can go through all the ups and downs and feel united in your exercise journey and the new path you are on. You'll likely share some laughs and, most importantly, support each other.

In addition to the psychological benefits and specific health goals, partner workouts are motivating for competitive individuals. Friendly competition can help workout buddies push each other. Especially for those further along their fitness journey, some hard-hitting competition may be exactly what is needed to take the workouts a step further and push outside of a comfort zone.

Exercise inspiration also develops from variety. When working out with a partner, there are many creative ways to put a new spin on familiar or favorite exercises. Who knew you could use your partner as a modified rowing machine or an agility marker? Variety increases enjoyment, decreases monotony, and challenges both partners. For these reasons, and many more listed in this chapter, partner workouts are a great way to join forces and tackle exercise with a fresh and fun approach.

CHAPTER 2

Foundations of Partner Training

Designing an effective exercise plan for partner workouts requires an understanding of the components of fitness, program design, movement, and performance training; an awareness of the various training principles; and identifying how to train to improve movement.

Whether you are an athlete or simply maintaining health goals, moving well day to day is paramount.

When it comes to exercise science and movement, there is a great deal written on training methodologies. In its simplest form, we train how we live. If we consider our day-to-day tasks, we are either moving or not. When we are not moving, we are in various stationary positions such as standing, sitting, crouching, or lying down. We may also be holding something weighted. Standing in line at the grocery store with an infant in one arm and a basket of groceries in the other is an example of a weighted stationary position.

As we move through our world, regardless if we are carrying something, we do so in different directions; at varying speeds; within changing or set movement patterns; at assorted angles, heights, and planes; and across different surfaces. Our movement patterns are changing all the time. For example, sprinting to catch the bus with a heavy backpack while trying to twist and maneuver through a crowd on an uneven sidewalk is reflective of real life, as is playing sports where we may be running, stopping, twisting, dodging, catching, ducking, hitting, balancing, shooting, or swinging in a match or game. Whether it is day-to-day living or structured activities, training only one fitness component, one or two selected body parts, or a single skill is never an ideal approach because it doesn't mimic true movement patterning. We must exercise and train how we live and play.

With that in mind, we must also train the secondary or performance-based components, in addition to cardiovascular conditioning, muscular and strength training, and flexibility training. These performance-based skills such as agility, balance, and speed training are necessary for day-to-day functioning and improved fitness.

Although these skills fall into a separate category and could be trained in isolation, they are often movements that are part of other exercises.

In a lunge, for example, having better balance will improve the ability to execute the movement pattern, both stationary and in motion. Training the muscles in a lunge through isolation and in compound exercises, and adding balance training as a separate component, helps to improve the overall execution of the lunge.

Performance-Based Components of Fitness

Performance-based components of fitness, also referred to as secondary or skill-related components (Magal and Scheinowitz 2018), differ from the primary training anchors that improve physical well-being. However, the secondary components are still important and are involved in all aspects of movement and activity, and are required for us to move through our daily lives.

- Balance is the ability to hold a specific body position in either a stationary or dynamic movement situation (Can-Fit-Pro 2010). In partner workouts, some of the exercises require one partner to be balanced while the other partner is doing an activity. To balance well, there needs to be concentration, focus, and a strategy such as reconnecting with the core or focusing on a specific spot on the floor. In addition, poor balance can also reflect weak muscles. Getting strong and staying fit will improve one's balance.

- Coordination is the ability to use the senses, such as sight and hearing, together with the body parts to perform tasks smoothly and accurately (Magal and Scheinowitz 2018). Some people are, or at least appear to be, more coordinated than others. Working with a partner requires many coordinated efforts to make an exercise a success. If this is not a strong skill for you or your partner, modify the move as needed and increase the amount of communication. Stating aloud what we are doing, while we are doing it—for example, saying, "out-out-in-in" while performing a footwork drill—often creates a greater mind–body connection.

- Agility is the ability to change body position with speed and accuracy (Magal and Scheinowitz 2018). Many of the cardio drills in partner workouts are focused on improving agility. Because agility occasionally requires coordination, starting slowly and mastering the footwork before adding speed can lead to a more successful outcome.

- Reaction time is the time elapsed to respond to a specific stimulus such as catching a ball or avoiding tripping over a log (Can-Fit-Pro 2010). A hockey player in a face-off situation must react and vie for the advantage between the time a referee blows the whistle and the puck is dropped. Each element has a set amount of time associated with the movement: from hearing the whistle, seeing the puck drop, waiting for it to hit the ice, and simultaneously responding. Many sports require quick reaction time. To train reaction time, incorporate various drills in which your partner responds to a command or catches a ball. For example, in a shuffling drill, cues such as "right, left, forward, or back" test how fast you and your partner can move in the specified direction.

• Speed is the ability to perform a movement in a short period of time (Magal and Scheinowitz 2018). With training, speed can be improved. Genetically, we have variations in the amount and function of different types of muscle fibers, which includes slow-twitch muscle fibers (type I) and fast-twitch type IIa and type IIb. The different muscle fibers in the body are classified by how they produce energy (Dintiman and Ward 2003). Therefore, the fibers can be trained using specific exercises designed to create energy and generate force. In a simple way, we can train based on our focus activity. Distance athletes have more slow-twitch muscle fiber whereas sprinters have more fast-twitch muscle fiber. It is, however, important to note that slow-twitch fibers can't be changed to fast-twitch fibers, but most of the intermediate fast-twitch type IIa fibers can be converted into faster-twitch type IIb fibers (Dintiman and Ward 2003). In simple terms—train fast, be fast.

• Power is the ability or rate at which one can perform work (Magal and Scheinowitz 2018). "Work, measured in joules, is a product of force and distance ($W = F \times D$)" (McCall 2019, p. 2). Moving a mass a distance requires muscular force (McCall 2019). Imagine a dumbbell biceps curl. The force is created in two ways: the muscles are challenged to produce greater magnitudes of force to move a heavy dumbbell or a lighter dumbbell is moved at a much faster rate or acceleration (McCall 2019). Power is measured in watts and is a product of force and velocity ($P = F \times V$). Moving a mass faster generates greater power. Adding power-based exercises to a partner workout will increase the intensity and complexity of many of the exercises. And if both partners are ready for that, it is a good way to train across all ages and demographics. We also need to be powerful every day. Basic functional movements like climbing the stairs or getting up and out of a chair require power. When we rise out of a chair, we are lifting our body weight with velocity. With that in mind, a training regime shouldn't focus on strength, speed, or power training alone, but should include all three.

• Mental focus is the ability to concentrate during exercise to improve training (Dintiman and Ward 2003), creating a mind–body connection. As a trainer, I often use the phrase, "think first and move second." This cue prompts clients or athletes to think about how they are positioned, the goal of the movement, how the muscles will respond, and what to do—all within a couple of seconds—before actually performing the exercise. Mental focus also allows you to get into the flow and enjoy the psychological and physical benefits that follow.

Programming for Success

Programming for success takes into consideration all the needs of an effective partner workout. This includes but is not limited to goal setting, program design, exercise selection, and more. Planning a workout is similar to following a recipe. As any successful baker knows, preparing and baking a cake with precision and care will result in a lighter and tastier confection. If you don't follow a recipe and just throw the ingredients into a bowl and hope for the best, chances are it will be a flop. Similarly, not making a workout plan and doing whatever exercise you feel like, or always doing the identical routine, will end in poor results. A step-by-step training plan, like using a recipe, is exactly what is needed for a successful partner workout.

Goal setting is step one. In baking, it's similar to deciding whether you want to make a chocolate or a vanilla cake. Once decided, the recipe is chosen, ingredients are gathered, and cooking utensils and equipment are set up. Then the recipe is followed line by line. Skipping steps, adding too much or too little of anything, or cranking up the oven beyond the required temperature may result in a dry or inedible cake. With fitness, we follow an exercise recipe. We select the exercises, choose the equipment, decide how many reps and sets to do, and determine how often to work out. A positive outcome in training, just like in baking, requires planning, preparation, action, and follow-up.

Exercise Selection

After goal setting, exercise selection is one of the most important variables when designing a program. Muscles get stronger when they are stressed and then adapt to the stressor. With that in mind, it is important to balance exercise choices to ensure that they don't favor certain muscles over others. Not doing so could cause muscular imbalances and lead to potential injury.

When choosing exercises, select ones with movement patterns that require greater integrations and muscle coordination. When multiple muscles fire together, they generate the forces needed for joint movement. Multijoint exercises that involve more than one joint or muscle group, as compared to isolation or single-joint movements that work one muscle or joint at a time, are preferred. Getting stronger is achieved when you focus on patterns that use more muscles. Squatting, lunging, hinging, pushing, pulling, and rotating are all movements that activate the major muscle groups in the lower body, upper body, and core. Training many of these foundational movements also corresponds with the movements we perform in everyday life.

Depending on the source you refer to, there are approximately nine identified foundational movement patterns. These include squat, lunge, hinge, push, pull, rotate, plank, lift, and gait. When we drop our keys on the ground and bend over to pick them up, that's a hinge. If your child is crying, you lower down to pick them up with a squat and lift. Reaching from the front to the back seat of your car to grab your gym bag requires your body to rotate. Slamming the trunk is a push, and reining in your dog as it chases a cat requires a pull. Everything you do in day-to-day life is a movement pattern or a series of movements.

Another variable in exercise selection is considering exercises that use larger-muscle groups. The use of larger muscles stimulates a greater aerobic response than exercises that focus on small-muscle groups. The body produces increased force when more muscles are activated, and this generates a greater work response. In turn, the increased muscle-fiber stimulus circulates a greater oxygen demand across the body in comparison to a smaller demand produced from less muscle-fiber stimulus (Langton and King 2018). A greater metabolic response provides additional benefits to training.

Other considerations for exercise selection are based on balancing movements around the joints. For example, working the hip joint through extension is complemented by working hip flexion. A biceps curl is balanced by training a triceps extension. It's also important to train the back of the body as well as the front. You are not only training the "mirror" muscles (i.e., the ones you can see in the mirror), but all of them.

Intensity

Another decision to make in exercise programming is intensity level. Intensity refers to the amount of weight or resistance used for strength training. The resistance chosen is based on individual needs, the type of exercise, and the number of reps. The goal is to overload the muscle so that adaptations and a metabolic response occur. When more weight is lifted, fewer reps are required to get the desired mechanical and metabolic response. If less weight is lifted, more reps are needed to get a similar response. However, in partner workouts, many of the exercises use body weight and don't require an external load or weight. You or your partner's weight is constant and doesn't change in an exercise session. With that in mind, intensity variations that make the exercise more challenging are modified through joint angles or body positions. For example, when performing the partner leg press in chapter 6, the exercise is easier when both partners are lying flat on the floor. When the hips are lifted at a 45-degree angle, the same exercise becomes much more challenging; its intensity has increased.

Rating of Perceived Exertion

Monitoring exercise intensity can be done in many ways. A heart rate strap, fitness tracker, or smartwatch can track metrics, such as heart rate, steps taken, activity minutes, sleep, calories, and even oxygen levels. Gadgets aside, the simplest way to monitor intensity is through perceived exertion. Often an individual's perception of exercise intensity (how hard they feel they are working) correlates very highly with their physiological response of heart rate, breathing rate, and cardiovascular and muscular fatigue. Using a very simple scale of 1-5 plus descriptors, you and your partner can rate exercise intensity from very easy to very hard. An RPE of 1 is very easy, 2 is easy, 3 moderate, 4 hard, and 5 is very hard. Notably, with time and training, an individual's RPE for the same exercise can change (decrease). This is a benefit of the training effect.

Repetitions

A repetition or "rep" is defined as "a single, individual action of movement at a joint or a series of joints that involves three phases of muscle action: muscle lengthening, a momentary pause, and muscle shortening" (McCall 2018). Reps and intensity often go hand in hand. If resistance is high (i.e., using a heavy weight) the number of repetitions that can be completed to momentary muscle fatigue is much less than if the resistance is light. Reps can also be time-based and centered around the amount that can be completed within a set amount of time. In partner workouts, most of the exercises are rep-based. However, there are a few exercises that complement a time-based approach, particularly when friendly competition comes into play.

Sets

When you finish a number of repetitions or complete the exercise within a specified amount of time, that is defined as a set. Sets are often bookmarked with a rest interval between each one. The total number of sets in an exercise sequence or workout is determined by the exercise goals and the amount of time available.

Tempo

Tempo is the speed of movement in an exercise and varies along the continuum from slow to fast. Throughout the partner workout exercise catalog, regressions and progressions are often made according to the speed at which a move is completed. Sometimes a fast movement makes an exercise harder, but it can also make it easier if momentum comes into play. Tempo is interchangeable based on the movement.

Another way to describe the tempo of an exercise is time under tension (TUT). Time under tension is defined as "the length of time muscle fibers are under mechanical tension from a resistance-training exercise" (McCall 2019). Like intensity, it affects mechanical and metabolic overload (McCall 2019).

Frequency

Frequency is the number of workouts completed over time. The client's stage of training (beginner to advanced) and an individual's or partners' programming goals will determine how often to schedule weekly or monthly workouts. Finding the correct workout frequency balance will lead to greater results. A new exerciser may be more comfortable scheduling fewer workouts initially, even though it is possible to exercise every day depending on program design. But scheduling too few workout sessions for a regular exerciser might lead to a plateau, and too many workouts could cause burnout. Frequency can fluctuate depending on several factors and is not always a constant; however, a consistent schedule is beneficial in partner workouts.

Exercise Order

Exercise order is an important variable in program design. The following suggestions are recommendations from ACSM that help support building an overall workout plan (Langton and King 2018).

Large-Muscle Groups Before Small-Muscle Groups

Training the large-muscle groups first is beneficial because it better prepares the body for other upcoming exercises. It is also a good way to warm up and get the muscles ready to go. Getting them fired up is advantageous for performing the exercises in the rest of the program.

Compound Exercises Before Isolation

Another term for compound exercises is multijoint movements. Compound exercises should be performed before single-joint, or isolation, exercises. A lunge and a push-up are good examples of compound exercises. Both the lunge and the push-up are exercises that engage multiple muscles across multiple joints. A calf raise and a chest fly are examples of isolation exercises. The lunge exercise engages muscles around the hip, knee, and ankle, while only the ankle joint is involved in the calf raise. Performing the lunge prior to the calf raise ensures the proper neuromuscular recruitment of the multijoint muscles and doesn't cause unbalanced activation of certain muscles. The smaller-muscle groups are often supporting players in a movement. If they are prefatigued, they won't be as effective in subsequent movements, which could compromise the quality of the movement and the overall training effect.

Alternating Push–Pull

For muscles to function effectively, they require a certain amount of rest between exercises. Alternating upper body pushing exercises with pulling exercises is a preferred way to balance a program because it allows maximal recovery time for the muscle groups between sets. An upper body training program that includes push-ups, chest press, rows, and pull-ups would not be best performed in that order. For better results, alternate pull-ups with push-ups and then rows and chest press. This alternates a pushing exercise with a pulling exercise instead of two pushing or two pulling exercises back-to-back. Alternating also improves circulatory response by increasing circulatory system adaptation. Instead of blood pooling in one location, it is diverted from one active muscle group to another active muscle group, as in the case with the pull-up to the push-up (Langton and King 2018).

Alternating Lower Body With Upper Body Exercises

A workout program that alternates lower body with upper body exercises is an excellent method for designing a full body workout. Full body workouts are especially valuable when clients are short on time and want to get more done in less time. Similar to the push–pull design, alternating the lower and upper body allows for maximum recovery time between muscle groups. Alternating squats with rows allows the lower body time to recover while the row is performed and vice versa. The longer recovery time improves the amount of force that can be generated in the next set and, in turn, improves the quality and overall performance of the muscle activation.

Explosive Actions and Power Lifts Before Basic Strength and Single-Joint Exercises

Power lifts such as a clean and jerk, or plyometrics such as an explosive box jump should be performed prior to other isolation or compound stationary exercises (Langton and King 2018). A great amount of power is required to generate these movement patterns, so prefatiguing the muscles necessary to do these types of moves is not ideal. These exercises also require a great deal of coordination, timing, and concentration. Performing them when tired can increase the risk of injury and may affect overall performance.

Weak Before Strong

It is easy to gravitate to the exercise that we do well and to train only the muscles that are strong. Prioritizing weaker muscles and movements first, by focusing on them earlier in the workout, provides the focus and the attention they need (Langton and King 2018). It also produces a more balanced body overall, which will benefit all movements.

High Intensity Before Low Intensity

If going "full out" is the goal, doing high-intensity work first should be the priority, especially when the body and the mind are fresh. Being able to totally focus one's effort will make a difference in the training effect. Also the body is better able to perform when it is not fatigued and hindered, or compromised in effort, coordination, or focus (Langton and King 2018).

Putting It All Together

Once the theoretical foundation of designing a partner workout has been explored, it is time to put theory into action. Each workout can be broken down into three main parts: the warm-up, which is the precursor to the upcoming workout; the main segment, which is the basis for the workout; and the cool-down and stretch to conclude.

Warm-Up

Before starting any exercise program, a warm-up is beneficial to prepare the body and the mind for the upcoming workout. Preparing correctly will improve the quality of the overall workout experience and decrease the risk of injuries. The warm-up also mentally prepares an exerciser for the workout. After a busy day of working or running around, immediately jumping into a workout session may only lead to a disorganized workout. The mind is just as important as the body when it comes to exercise.

The easiest way to prepare for any exercise session or activity is to do the activity of choice or the foundational exercises at a much gentler pace or easier intensity. Going for a run shouldn't amount to opening the door and taking off at breakneck speed. The intended exerciser most likely starts with a walk, then a jog, transitions into some stretches that focus on the muscles used for running, returns to the jog, and finally increases the pace and intensity to run.

By starting slow, the muscles, ligaments, joints, various structures, cardiorespiratory system, and other body parts have a chance to adapt to the imposed stimulus and rev up the neuromuscular messaging and energy needed to prepare for movement. There is a gradual increase in body temperature, which is stimulated by responses such as increased heart rate, blood flow, and breathing rate. The body starts to move better with enhanced nerve transmission telling the muscles what to do and how to do it. It is like starting an old car. Instead of revving it up high, we give it a little gas and gently ease it out of the garage.

The main functions of a warm-up can be broken down into movement rehearsal, increased body temperature with cardiorespiratory response, mobility training (moving in various directions and at different speeds), and functional and mental preparation. Stretching before warming up is counterproductive and can increase the risk of injuries. Be sure to move the joints through their range of motion to gently lengthen the muscles and surrounding connective tissues. Save the holding stretches for the end of the workout.

Many of the cardio drills in the partner workouts can be adapted for the warm-up. A running drill can be done at a light jog, a jumping drill can be done as a squat to press, and a burpee can be done in slow motion. Be creative and modify intensity.

Essential to an effective warm-up is connecting with your partner. Being in sync with them will make the more challenging combinations later in the workout easier to coordinate and complete. An exercise like the lunge and press in chapter 6 combines a foundational, multijoint exercise. The hand press then release requires concentration and communication, which stimulates the body and the mind.

Workout

The main part of an exercise program is composed of the workout. Within chapters 11 to 16 are different sample partner workouts with varying focus areas. Whether it is a HIIT workout, a circuit format, sports-specific, or a beginner exercise plan, each provides you with ideas of how to effectively train with your partner.

Cool-Down and Stretch

The cool-down is the cousin to the warm-up. Similar but somewhat different, it is the reverse of the warm-up phase. After the main part of the workout is complete, allow the heart and breathing rate to gradually return to preexercise levels. This is called the postcardio or postworkout phase. Finally, always leave time to stretch. Stretching when the body is still warm is optimal and preferred. Hold each position for a minimum of 30 to 60 seconds, breathe normally, relax into the stretch, and enjoy the relaxation time with your partner. Chapter 10 provides a list of flexibility exercises to try with your partner.

CHAPTER 3

Training Equipment and Workout Space

One of the many benefits of partner training is the option to use small pieces of equipment, or in some cases, no equipment at all. Ease of use, portability, cost, availability, and effectiveness are all factors when considering whether a piece of equipment will add to or detract from a particular partner exercise. Fitness professionals understand that equipment is chosen judiciously and its use affects its value. When we add load to movement, we challenge the body to adapt to the new stimulus. This adaptation creates stronger muscles, improves mobility and stability, strengthens the core, and assists body functions in everyday activities.

Because various small pieces of equipment weigh the same amount, an interchangeable approach to finding the best one for specific exercises is recommended. A 10-pound (4.5 kg) medicine ball weighs the same as a 10-pound (4.5 kg) dumbbell, kettlebell, or weight plate. But tossing a kettlebell to your partner, which is a hard piece of equipment with an odd handle shape, would not be the ideal choice in a throwing exercise. A medicine ball or plyo ball is specifically designed for most passing drills and is the better and safer choice.

When selecting the right equipment, it is important to choose correctly and consider risk versus benefit. Avoid adding equipment to an exercise just for the sake of it; make sure there is a purpose behind the choice of equipment. Each piece of small equipment has a particular function that is more conducive to certain types of exercise and movements than others.

Additional benefits to small pieces of equipment include cost and accessibility. Most are relatively inexpensive, especially in comparison to bulky and large exercise machines. An exercise band can be purchased for under 20 dollars and is available in most sports equipment or fitness stores. They can even be found in some pharmacies and big box stores. Resistance bands have multiple uses, are easy to store, and travel well. A band can be thrown in a sports bag or suitcase and easily used at different locations whether it's at the gym, at home, or on vacation.

Lastly, small equipment can be used as an effective buffer between partners. Some partnerships will be new, and not everyone will be comfortable being close to or touching each other. Holding onto a resistance

At Home Equipment Options

No equipment? No problem. Try some of these options:

Traditional	Alternative
Dumbbells	Canned goods, water bottles, milk jugs or paint cans (upcycled and filled with sand or water)
Barre	Sturdy chair, counter
Bands	Nylons, upcycled leggings
Straps	Neckties, belts, robe ties
Mats	Towels, folded sheet, blanket
Gliding discs	Paper plates (plastic)
Small ball	Soccer ball, volleyball
Workout bench	Sturdy chair, bench seat without a back

band, tossing a medicine ball, or squatting using a stability ball while back-to-back creates a comfortable barrier between partners. It is like creating an equipment security bubble.

Elastic Resistance Training Equipment (Bands and Tubing)

Bands and tubing fall under the category of elastic resistance training equipment. There are many types of elastic resistance training tools with the most common grouped under the class of flat bands or tubing. Tubing is often open-ended (not looped), covered or uncovered, and available with or without handles. They are also available in varied resistances. Flat bands are offered looped or open-ended, are sold in various lengths, and are also available in different thicknesses that provide varying resistance.

There are many benefits to elastic resistance equipment. Using a band or tube, increases in resistance provide a progressive stimulus to the muscle (Freytag 2020; Silva Lopes et al. 2019; Harvard Medical School 2019; Stoppani 2020; Walker 2016; Iversen et al. 2017; Elite Performance Institute 2020). Single- or multiple-joint movements can be trained using resistance bands for more efficient and functional exercises. Unlike training with weighted equipment, elastic resistance does not rely on gravity to assist or challenge muscles. When completing a biceps curl with dumbbells, the biceps muscles work against gravity in the concentric or lifting phase of the curl, and gravity assists in the eccentric or lowering phase of the exercise.

In contrast, the length a band stretches will determine the resistance. At each stage of elongation, the resistance relative to pounds increases. As the band moves away from the attachment point, the resistance increases anywhere from 25 percent elongation up to greater than 250 percent elongation depending on the composition of the band. As the band moves closer to the anchor, shortening the elongation, the intensity decreases.

Elastic resistance training also offers many movement options for increased functional training, and multiple directions of motion for varied exercise possibilities. Speed and power training can be attempted safely and effectively because of the bands' elastic characteristics. For example, anchoring the band under one foot and performing a wood chop exercise by holding the opposite end of an unlooped band can be executed at various tempos from slow to fast, depending on the training focus. However, the same movement executed using a weighted dumbbell would need to be performed at a slower tempo, on both the concentric and eccentric phase of the movement. Based on Newton's first law, a mass in motion stays in motion with the same speed and in the same direction unless acted upon by an outside force (Hodanbosi 1996). Lifting and lowering a dumbbell could potentially cause a muscle injury if the motion is too fast, if the weight is too heavy, or if the momentum of the movement can't be stopped correctly. Using elastic resistance allows you to move the band at various speeds from the anchor point.

Prior to using a resistance band or tubing, always check the integrity of the material. The band should be free of nicks or tears. Any damage to the band may result in the band tearing midexercise and could cause injury to yourself or partner. Always replace damaged bands as necessary.

Most elastic resistance training equipment comes in various resistance levels, from light to strong. Elastic resistance manufacturers will use different tubes or band colors to distinguish the pounds of resistance. In general, lighter-colored bands tend to be easier to use and considered lower resistance. For example, SPRI and TheraBand resistance bands use a resistance scale with light-colored bands being the easiest and dark-colored bands being more challenging.

When using the flat band or resistance tubing, maintain proper wrist alignment while holding the band and ensure the anchoring position of the band is based on the best line of pull for the chosen exercise. When securing the band, check that it is fastened correctly to any attachment points, especially if you or your partner are standing on the band or wrapping it around a body part.

The setup for anchoring the band depends on the exercise and may require the handle through the handle, standing on it, a wrap around the feet, attaching it to a secure structure, or working with a partner (see table 3.1). A good rule of thumb when working with any resistance tubing is to keep some tension on the band, both in the concentric and eccentric phases of movements, and avoid letting the band snap back to the starting position (Page and Ellenbecker 2020).

Table 3.1   Anchoring the Band

Standing on one end of the band and holding the other end in the hand	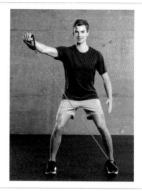
Standing on the band, holding both handles, offset under one foot or centered under both feet	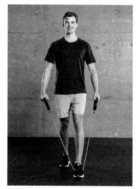 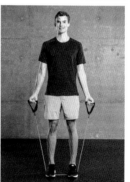
Wrapping the band around both feet in a seated position	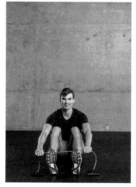 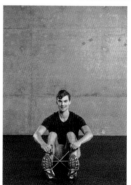
Holding the band overhead	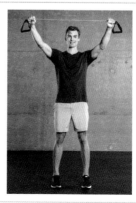

Center anchor with multiple bands	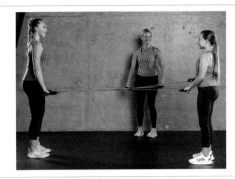
Partner holds the band from behind	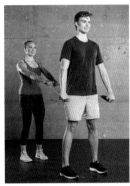
Partner holds the band from the front	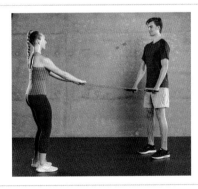

Medicine Balls

The medicine ball is an easy piece of equipment to add to any partner workout. When it is used correctly, it is both challenging and functional. It is also a fun training tool. Any time equipment inspires play, like tossing a ball or jumping on a rebounder, the exercise is less like working out and more like recreation.

Working out with a medicine ball is not new. The first recorded photograph of a weighted exercise ball was taken in 1866 with a Harvard fitness trainer. Even ancient Hippocrates was thought to have used one (Heffernan 2020). Today, fitness professionals, coaches, and home exercisers regularly integrate the medicine ball into their workouts.

There are many benefits to medicine ball training. It adds variety to a program, is inexpensive, is portable for both indoor and outdoor use, and can be used in strength and cardio circuits.

Choose an appropriately sized medicine ball for maximum benefit and safety. Choosing a medicine ball size depends on a number of factors including fitness level and overall strength. Medicine balls are available in a variety of dimensions and weigh from two pounds (1 kg) to over 22 pounds (10 kgs). There are a number of brands and types of balls available. Some are made of leather and don't bounce, others are inflatable and bouncy, some squish when dropped such as a plyo ball, some are full of sand and flatten when they hit the floor such as a slam ball, while others come with various textured surfaces. The ball's intended use will determine the selection. Medicine balls are relatively inexpensive and can be purchased from sporting goods stores and big box retail stores.

When exercising with a medicine ball, choose a starting weight that will accommodate the weaker partner. Medicine balls can provide intensity options for any given exercise when you outline progressions using various stages. Using the principles of progressive overload, gradually increase the repetitions, resistance level or lever length of holds, or add advanced exercises to challenge each individual appropriately. The harder, faster, and greater distance a ball is thrown, the more muscle fibers recruited, contracting eccentrically to decelerate the ball. Because eccentric contractions are generally associated with muscle soreness, start medicine ball training with concentric contractions. For example, your partner could begin by catching only, instead of catching and throwing, the medicine ball.

Medicine balls can add progressive overload to an exercise sequence in numerous ways. The first option is to hold the medicine ball close to the torso in a stable position while performing foundational movements. In a squat exercise, the medicine ball is held close to the chest. To increase the challenge, concurrently take the medicine ball through a complementary or counterbalancing range of motion. Using the squat example, the medicine ball is held away from the body at shoulder level.

As you progress the squat range of motion downward, pull the medicine ball and arms toward the abdomen and then return the ball back to the starting position as you lift from the squat. In the third example, the medicine ball is released at the extension of a dynamic movement. Squat with the ball extended in front of the body at shoulder level, lowering the legs and arms, and then lift, releasing the medicine ball at the top, tossing the ball with control and catching it or passing it to your partner.

Tossing and catching a weighted ball is a form of plyometric training. We often think of plyometrics as jumping and don't always translate this style of training to the upper body. Plyometrics are an exercise that "involves a stretch of the muscle-tendon unit immediately followed by a shortening of the muscle unit" (Chu and Myer 2013). This rapid muscle lengthening and shortening cycle is key to plyometrics exercises and enables a muscle to reach maximum strength in a short time. It often involves repeated, rapid eccentric and concentric movements to increase muscular power (Chu and Myer 2013). Upper body plyometrics often include throwing, passing, and catching movements. These upper body plyometric movements build and improve the explosive power in the back, chest, shoulders, and arms (Australian Fitness Academy 2019). Dynamic and vertical ball training increases torso strength and endurance allowing the midsection to better absorb impact forces. Medicine ball training can be very effective in partner workouts and can help improve upper body strength and power, core conditioning, coordination, and reaction time.

Bodyweight Training

Occasionally, the best exercise equipment is no equipment at all. Bodyweight training uses your own body mass (upper and lower regions and the core) as resistance for various individual and partner exercises. Additional equipment such as dumbbells or other weighted tools is unnecessary to add load to a movement, and emphasis is placed on doing exercises using only the body.

Bodyweight training is a do-anywhere, do-it-all training platform. For years, personal trainers and fitness companies recognized the benefits of streamlining multiple workout equipment options with a "less is more" approach. TRX suspension training even coined the slogan, "make your body your machine," highlighting the benefits of using one's own body weight as the resistance in addition to their suspension strap. Common bodyweight exercises include the push-up, squat, lunge, abdominal curl, and plank, plus others and many variations on these movements.

Bodyweight training benefits traditional fitness goals like strength, speed, power and endurance, as well as functional movement patterns like balance and coordination. Performing a customary squat combined with a one-legged bounding move requires strength, power, balance, and coordination. The exercise becomes more functional as it becomes multilayered.

Likewise, day-to-day movements incorporate multiple planes of movement. The three planes of movement include the sagittal, frontal, and transverse planes. The sagittal plane divides the body into right and left halves with an imaginary line. Any movement that is parallel to this line occurs in the sagittal plane. For example, exercises composed primarily of flexion and extension joint movements are sagittal (Payne 2019). Examples include a biceps curl in which there is flexion and extension at the wrist, elbow, and shoulder, or a lunge, in which the movement is forward or back. There is no side-to-side movement in these types of exercises.

The frontal plane includes lateral and medial support and represents the body being divided into front and back halves. To visualize frontal planes, imagine that the body is pressed between two plates of glass, creating a space where the body can only move from side to side, but it can't move forward or backward (Payne 2019). Any lateral, side-to-side movement parallel to this imaginary line occurs in the frontal plane. Examples of movements in the frontal plane are the side arm raise, side lunge, side bend, and jumping jack.

The third plane is called the transverse plane. When we consider movements like spinal or limb rotations, the motion divides the body into top and bottom halves (Payne 2019). However, imagine an axis that extends vertically from the top of the head and through the spine. Movement occurs around this axis. Twisting the spine or rotating a limb away from or to the center of the body works the transverse plane. This includes internally and externally rotating our limbs toward or away from the midline, respectively. Shoulder and hip movements also fall under the transverse plane category. When the arms are extended out to the sides at shoulder height, and we bring them together, we are working in the transverse plane; hip abduction or adduction movements are also transverse plane movements. It would appear that we should be in the sagittal plane, but because of the rotation that happens at the hip and shoulder joints, these types of movements are in the transverse plane.

In day-to-day life, we move in all three planes. We climb stairs (sagittal plane), stretch our arms out to the side (frontal plane), and toss our gym bag over our shoulder before we head into the studio (transverse plane). With that in mind, and as discussed earlier, we should train how we move. This is a benefit of bodyweight training, especially as we program with a variety of movements. In contrast, when using the selectorized-style of exercise equipment (i.e., weight machines), the body is often placed in a position that works only one plane of motion. On a hamstring curl machine, lying prone and moving a stationary weight toward your glutes is working in the sagittal plane. This movement does strengthen the hamstrings; however, there are greater benefits to strengthening more muscles and moving in various directions at one time. When running around a tennis court, we use the hamstring muscles. However, we also need to strengthen the other muscles that connect the hip and the knee as well as the upper body and core. Instead of the hamstring curl machine,

Setting Up Your Workout Space

With more of us choosing to train from home, creating a home gym is a great solution. When trying to find that "just right" space, consider the following:

• *Location.* Finding the ideal spot to train may be one of the biggest challenges. A spare room would be ideal, but not always possible. With that in mind, space-creativity is needed. At a minimum, you and your partner should be two arm-lengths apart when standing side by side. When facing each other, you should each be able to hold a straight-legged, arm-extended plank without touching. Forward jumping or using two resistance bands may require a bit more creativity or may not always be possible in a space. Exercise options or modifications need to be explored.

• *Flooring.* Ideally hardwood, laminate, or tile flooring would be best because it is much easier to keep clean and easier to exercise on. Shoes should be worn with most of the exercises in partner workouts. Carpet tends to grip shoes and is not as sanitary. If your space is carpeted, consider purchasing exercise-type flooring that can be placed in the space and removed if necessary.

• *Storage.* Equipment storage is crucial in a small space. Keeping the floor clutter-free is an important safety consideration. Dumbbell tree-style holders can be purchased and keep weights off the floor. Other options include purchasing adjustable dumbbells that can be made heavier or lighter by clicking the weights in or out, all within a single dumbbell. Wall hooks can hold lighter items such as straps, bands, and tubing, and a ceiling net can house lighter stability or yoga balls. Mats can also be hung up or rolled and stored in a corner. Medicine balls can be placed in a sturdy bin. A bench can be used for step-ups or other exercises, and can also store equipment underneath.

• *Airflow.* A cool workout area is ideal. Air conditioning, or a space with a window and good airflow is important. Having access to fresh air is a preferable option. If that's not possible, consider purchasing an air filtration and fan system.

• *Add-Ons.* A bright space is energizing, and natural light is ideal. With any lighting, choose LED because it doesn't increase room temperature. A full-length mirror is helpful for analyzing movement and making corrections. A mirror can be portable or hung permanently on a wall. A compact speaker with Bluetooth linked to a smartphone is a good option for music. Background music is always motivating and energizes a space. If you are painting a designated workout space, choose cool colors and avoid warm colors that can make a space feel hot. Keep a water bottle and a workout towel handy.

performing a side-to-side resistance band bounding move with your partner works more than one muscle group in various planes of motion. A multiplanar, multimuscle approach to training will better benefit the whole body and improve how we move through the world each day.

Anyone can perform bodyweight training exercises, but there are some best practices to consider. The first is to focus on proper alignment. If you build a home with a faulty foundation, eventually your entire house will have significant structural issues. The same goes for your body. Focus on proper alignment that initiates from the feet all the way through to the top of the head. Next, the core must always be active. A sloppy core does not give the body the stability it needs to move well. Think of the core as the powerhouse that surrounds our body like a muscular girdle. If the core is weak, all movements will be compromised. Finally, the mind plays a powerful role in movement and muscle engagement. Electromyography (EMG) studies have shown that when we focus on the muscles that we are working during the exercise versus just going through the motion of the movement, there is a greater training effect. An EMG device measures the very small electrical impulses that occur when the muscle fibers are stressed (Raineri 2015).

Movement and muscle focus in bodyweight training becomes imperative when there is no external load challenging the muscles. A preferred cue for better results is, "Think first, move second," implying that you should focus on what you are about to do before you start.

Workout Space

When working out with a partner, space becomes a crucial consideration. You might even think of it as an extra piece of equipment because having the right amount of space is important to perform all exercises safely and effectively.

Partners may choose to work out at each other's homes, outdoors, at a training center, or at a gym. To determine how much space is needed, first decide on the type of training plan or exercises you will be doing. A cardio-focused workout requires enough room for two people to perform expansive movements such as jumping or skipping, and requires a cool, ventilated area. Strength-focused workouts may require less space, but if there is equipment involved, room size and storage must be considered. Throwing a medicine ball with your partner will require more open space and more focus. No one wants a medicine ball accidentally thrown through a window, or the family heirloom smashed by a wayward dumbbell. For more specifics on setting up your space, see the Setting Up Your Workout Space sidebar.

CHAPTER 4

Partner Roles and Goals

Successful partnerships start by connecting with the right person. Regardless of physical differences or environmental limitations, partners need to be in sync and engaged in the overall process. Additional strategies such as program design and creating workable training spaces only add positively to the partnership.

Choosing a Partner

Partnerships often materialize organically with friends or family members choosing to exercise together. Certain partner pairings are more successful than others. Similar strength and fitness levels lend themselves to a physically successful partnership. But even if you're not perfectly matched, a mother–son, a grandfather–granddaughter, or a fit–unfit couple are all still potential partners. These combinations can be successful; they simply require modifications.

Regardless of similarities or differences, an overall desire to accomplish goals might be enough to overcome any physical asymmetries. The concept that a chain is only as strong as its weakest link is fitting when it comes to forecasting how to make any partnership thrive. Partners must always work together to increase the successful completion of each exercise, similar to making a pass–catch during a basketball game. A player will have a more difficult time scoring if a teammate can't pass the ball correctly.

Each partner has an incredibly important role in making the other more successful. Communication is key. Partners need to be able to talk to each other and share feedback. Both partners need to feel secure and confident enough to communicate not just how they are feeling, but steps to make the exercises easier, more challenging, or more comfortable. Asking questions like, "Is this too much pressure?" or, "Do you want to try a heavier medicine ball?" or even suggesting positioning cues such as, "We both need to focus on keeping our core engaged during this exercise," are all examples of feedback that can come from each partner, or from a personal trainer facilitating the session (see more information on personal training and partner workouts in the appendix of this book). Just like in any successful relationship, good communication is foundational.

Safe Training

Exercise always carries some inherent risk. To reduce some of that risk, follow these guidelines before starting your partner workouts.

- *Complete a physical activity readiness questionnaire* (PAR-Q; www. eparmedx.com). This is a precursor to starting any new exercise program and helps you identify potential health issues before you start. Make certain that you and your partner have received the green light from your health care provider.

- *Listen to your body.* Understand basic training principles, and always listen to the subtle and maybe not-so-subtle signals that your body sends. This means if something hurts, stop. Some discomfort associated with working out is generally okay, but pain is a feedback response that should never be ignored. If a movement or exercise hurts, stop and reevaluate. Modify, reposition, limit the range of motion, decrease the load, or stop all together.

- *Always start slow.* A new exercise program should be likened to running a marathon, not a sprint. Ease into your new training regime so that neither of you get burned out or become plagued by injuries.

- *Never jump into a workout without warming up.* Always warm up gradually and progressively for approximately five to eight minutes and follow the suggestions in chapter 2.

- *Before beginning, ensure that you and your partner have enough room to move.* Keep the area clear so you won't be hampered by furniture or trip over any equipment.

- *Stay cool and hydrated.* Overheating is not only uncomfortable, but it can be dangerous and impede the quality of your workout. Keep the room temperature cool and a water bottle handy. Take sips of water throughout the workout to stay hydrated.

- *Wear exercise-appropriate clothing.* Workout clothing should wick moisture, allow you to move easily, and be appropriate for some of the more "close up" partner exercises. Appropriate shoes are also recommended, and remove any jewelry that could catch on your partner.

- *Fuel up before exercise.* A light snack one to two hours before a workout will give you the energy needed to train and perform at your best. Refuel on a healthy snack of carbs and proteins within 30 minutes postworkout.

- *Be consistent and have a positive mindset.* Fostering regular exercise to become a habit is beneficial both physically and mentally. Set and stick to ruthless rituals. Schedule and commit to your workouts.

Having a positive mindset involves making every moment better than the last. Start with a great attitude and be ready. Be the best partner you can be.

- *Stretch.* Cool down gradually for approximately five minutes and set aside enough time to stretch. We can't move well if we can barely touch our toes or lift our hands over our head. Be sure to stretch the main muscles of the lower and upper body. For stretching ideas, refer to the exercises listed in chapter 10.

Virtual Partner Workouts

In-person partner workouts may not always be possible, so a virtual option is a perfect alternative. Zoom, Facetime, or Skype-type meetings allow you to be connected, even if you are physically apart. Whether you are a personal trainer taking a lead in the session, or partners scheduling their own workout, a little planning and preparation go a long way (see more information on personal training and partner workouts in the appendix of this book). Try some of these tips to help make a remote partner session more successful.

- *Technology.* First decide on a technology that both partners have available and are comfortable using. There is not a right or wrong option, but rather one that works best for everyone involved. Some streaming platforms are free, whereas others have a subscription fee. Research which option will work better.

- *Environment.* Similar to creating a training space when you are exercising together, the workout area matters. Make sure the space is clear of clutter, any required equipment is ready to go, there is proper ventilation, and the floor surface is appropriate.

If you are using a laptop, make sure the camera is positioned so that the whole body and all movements are in the frame. A smartphone will work, but it is small and more challenging to see the exercises properly.

- *Exercise choice.* When training virtually with a partner, choosing the correct exercises and modifying any partner-assisted or -resisted movements require some planning. Understandably, partner training is meant to be done with a partner, but in some situations virtually connecting is better than nothing. The easiest type of training plan in this situation is an alternating format. Partner A does exercise 1 and partner B does exercise 2 for a set number of reps or time, before switching. If an exercise requires a partner anchor, for example, when using a resistance band, find a secure alternative. A doorjamb designed to hold a resistance band or a strap can be purchased. A chair can be used to assist in an exercise like a pistol squat versus holding onto a partner's hand.

- *Fun.* Partners should plan for a few fun challenges between each other. For example, each partner could perform the same exercise for a set amount of time, such as burpees, and see who completes more. Mix up the challenges so each partner has a chance to out-do their workout buddy. Not a competitive partnership? No problem. Include simple and less intimidating challenges, such as balance exercises or agility work.

- *Expectations.* Virtual and online training is not perfect, but it continues to improve every day. When working from home—or working out at home—there seems to be a greater level of tolerance for the dog that runs through the meeting frame or the teen that calls incessantly in the middle of the workout. However, it is important to value your partner's time and minimize distractions that could take away from the training experience.

Partner Considerations

When choosing a partner, body composition (height and weight), ability (skill set), fitness level (beginner or advanced), goals (commitment), age, and drive should all be considered. But beyond the physical similarities, developing and nurturing a fun, supportive, and encouraging workout relationship is fundamental to a successful training partnership. Being like-minded with a positive approach to one's combined training goals is also advantageous, as is staying committed. Even in a "perfect match," if your partner doesn't show up or isn't engaged in the process, similarities or differences will no longer matter. Connect with a partner who is open to trying new workouts and motivated to put the effort into getting fit and healthy. Table 4.1 offers some ideas on how to make a new partner arrangement work for both of you.

Partnerships can benefit from respectful competition. It can be the extra push that motivates a person to try harder. Healthy competition can add variety and excitement to a predictable situation and strengthen bonds by becoming each other's cheerleaders. What isn't warranted is unhealthy competition. Winning at all costs or actively diminishing the efforts of your partner is futile. The goal is to better each other, not tear each other down. Choose a partner that suits your personality and training style by complementing you, or go out on a limb and find someone who will challenge and bring out your competitive side.

Accommodating Mismatched Partners

In some training situations, having an equally matched partner is not always possible or feasible. A couple working out together creates an ideal partnership based on their household circumstances. But it is not

Table 4.1   Increasing the Comfort With a New Workout Partner

Tips	Examples
Use a piece of equipment to act as a buffer between partners	Medicine ball, resistance band, stability ball, glider
Be cognizant of the positioning of the partners	Select side-by-side positions and limit face-to-face or other up-close positions
Make correct contact when adding partner resistance	Place the hands on your partner's boney spots (e.g., shoulder blade, hip bone) whenever possible
Break up the number of partner exercises	Alternate between a solo exercise and a partner exercise
Mix up the format	Set up stations, alternate between cardio and strength, work in tandem on the same or different exercises

necessarily a perfect match. Although they are very comfortable with each other, they may not be evenly matched physically. In this couple scenario, one partner may be shorter and more cardiovascular fit, and the other partner may be stronger and weigh much more.

With an uneven matchup, choosing the correct workout format and exercise combinations become an important program planning consideration. In this example, exercises that alternate from one partner to another may be a better option. For example, the stronger partner does 45 seconds of jumping jacks while the shorter partner performs push-ups, then they switch. The stronger partner transitions to the push-ups and the shorter partner does the jumping jacks. In the next set, the stronger partner performs bent-over rows with 30-pound weights and the wife skips, switching again after the designated time. But in this round, the shorter partner uses a 15-pound weight set. Both partners perform the same exercise, but at different loads and intensities.

In partner workouts with two evenly matched partners, format choice tends to be easier. Generally, any type of training plan will work and require minimal modifications. With mismatched partners, program consideration factors strongly into the workout equation. Bodyweight partner exercises, in which one partner is using the other partner for resistance, are not always ideal for partners that are very unevenly matched. For example, in a plank and push-up combination (see page 64), one partner holds a straight-arm plank while the other performs a push-up on the partner's back. This exercise would be too intense for the weaker partner, especially in holding the plank position.

Other partner mismatches may include one partner having an injury or chronic condition, differences in fitness levels, extremes in body composition, or varying degrees of commitment or drive. It doesn't mean the partnership won't work; it just requires additional planning, appropriate format choices, and modifying some of the exercises.

Partner Training With Children

Embodying a healthy and active lifestyle is the best gift you can give a child. Children and teens often use stimuli from the world around them to form opinions and establish thought processes early on about various concepts and actions.

As parents and caregivers, our actions often matter more than our words, and it is our subtle acts that can be the most powerful. Even if you never talk about the importance of exercise, when children see you doing it on a regular basis, they have established a connection.

Partner workouts with children and teens are an excellent way to connect with kids and engage in a fun workout that could possibly involve the entire family. Although not all exercises may be appropriate because of the age of the child, development stage, size difference, and overall ability, a great deal can be modified. The goal is not to perfect the exercise, but rather to be engaged and moving.

To get started, choose exercises that fall under the easy- to moderate-intensity levels, such as follow the leader (see page 130), which is interactive and fun, or try some of the less challenging cardio-focused moves. Children and young teens can better manage short-burst cardio exercise versus long duration sets. Using a piece of equipment is also a good option, especially tossing around a light medicine ball. Most kids are skilled at throwing activities. Lastly, if exercises are combined, such as the wide plank and agility footwork exercises in chapter 8, separate them into two. Mom does the plank and the son does the agility move, but he does not do the agility steps over the top of Mom's feet as originally designed.

Regardless of the age of the child, keep the workout short, lasting approximately 20 to 30 minutes. The goal is to have fun, be engaged, sweat a little, and then let kids move on to the next activity in their day. And who knows, if the workout feels fun and too short, they may ask for more. It becomes something they want to do, versus your driving it.

Goal Setting Together

Goal setting is an important first step in establishing short- and long-term targets, and setting personal and partner goals. Short-term goals represent the day-to-day and week-to-week planning that is necessary to achieve a long-term goal. For example, perhaps you and your partner

Quick Tips—Building Successful Partnerships

- Create trust.
- Ensure a strong foundation.
- Promote good communication.
- Modify exercises to meet the abilities of both partners.
- Apply the correct pressure, resistance, or support.
- Emphasize working together in a coordinated effort.

would like to participate in an outdoor endurance race that is happening nine months from the onset of your training. Simply signing up for an event won't cut it. Setting weekly goals, including the number of training days and the format to follow, provides direction and focus, and ensures you are both prepared for race day.

It is also important to set individual goals to define what you want to achieve personally. Individual goals may include aspirations to lose weight, get stronger, boost energy, stay healthy, or simply stay committed to an exercise regime. Both partner and individual goals can be aligned and relate to each other. Finishing in the top 20 in your age category at a race and getting stronger are mutually beneficial to you and your partner.

Step one is to bond with your partner. If this is a new connection, getting to know your partner is crucial to a successful training relationship. Discussing neutral topics, such as exercise experience or a favorite sport, is a great place to start. If you are training with someone familiar, the introduction phase is not necessary since you already have a preestablished relationship.

Step two is to pull out a calendar and choose an agreed-upon goal date to work toward. Initially stick with a four- to six-month long-term goal. If a goal is set too far in the future, goal attainment may be hampered by unrealistic timelines and a higher fail rate. Choose either an event (e.g., a race or activity) or something tangible and quantifiable (e.g., push-ups or fitting into your favorite jeans).

Even if partner training is for pure enjoyment, it is important to establish some goals. Goal setting is the glue that will keep the train on the tracks. As with any goal setting, be as specific as possible and establish a plan based on the SMART acronym: **S**pecific, **M**easurable, **A**ssignable, **R**ealistic, and **T**ime-related (Doran 1981). Goal setting guides the process, streamlines effort, and increases the overall success rate.

Once a long-term partner or team goal has been established, delve into individual goal setting. Ask yourself and each other questions that will help define your starting point and ideals moving forward.

- How would you rate your fitness level on a scale from 1 to 10 (1 not exercising and 10 extremely fit)?
- If you are not at your ideal fitness level, describe a time when you were.
- What helped you get fit during that time?
- What do each of you want to achieve?
- Is this a new goal or a goal you had in the past?
- How committed are each of you to the process?
- How often can you commit to working out?
- How can you make this a mutually beneficial process?

And the most important questions to ask when it comes to goal attainment is: "What stopped you from achieving your goal in the past, or what do you perceive to be the roadblock(s) to reaching your goal?" Breaking down roadblocks is almost as important as setting goals. We can often come up with a goal and a plan, but we don't usually determine or lean into what stopped us from being successful during previous attempts. For example, if your goal was to exercise three times per week by taking the 5:00 p.m. bootcamp class, and you only got to the gym once or twice a week, what happened? If it was because you always ended up working late or you were too tired by the end of the day, the roadblock is the time of day. Exercising before work may be the solution to the roadblock and could improve your chances of goal success.

After establishing a long-term team goal, individual goals, and a roadblock plan, focus on the how-to steps. Decide with your partner how many workouts you will do together and how many you will do separately. Based on the Physical Activity Guidelines for Americans, 2nd Edition, for "substantial health benefits, adults should do at least 150 minutes (2 hours and 30 minutes) to 300 minutes (5 hours) a week of moderate-intensity, or 75 minutes (1 hour and 15 minutes) to 150 minutes (2 hours and 30 minutes) a week of vigorous-intensity aerobic physical activity, or an equivalent combination of moderate- and vigorous-intensity aerobic activity. Preferably, aerobic activity should be spread throughout the week. Additional health benefits are gained by engaging in physical activity beyond the equivalent of 300 minutes (5 hours) of moderate-intensity physical activity a week. Adults should also do muscle-strengthening activities of moderate or greater intensity and that involve all major muscle groups on 2 or more days a week, as these activities provide additional health benefits" (USDHHS 2018).

To establish a training plan based on these recommendations, follow the well-established FITT-VP guidelines (frequency, intensity, time, type, volume, progression) that work best for you and your partner (DeSimone 2019). Frequency establishes how often to work out per week, ideally aiming to exercise on most days of the week, perhaps with at least one to two partner workouts. Intensity refers to how easy or hard to exercise. On a four workout per week rotation, for example, start by scheduling one easy, two moderate, and one challenging workout session, depending on your starting point. If an exercise regime is totally new, the workouts may all be easy to begin. For a length of time, vary it according to the intensity. On challenging cardio days, keep the workout shorter, approximately 30 minutes, and on easy days extend the workout duration to include strength and cardio work. The last T in FITT stands for type of workout. There are many types to follow and variety is important. Varying formats, mixing up equipment, or even changing the workout location will help avoid boredom. Lastly, VP refers to volume and progression. The volume of exercise—the product of frequency, intensity, and time—is fluid. For example, some days an exerciser may have less time to work out. In that case, an individual can increase a workout's intensity or include an

Personalizing a Fitness SWEAT

Businesses are familiar with the process of going through a SWOT analysis to determine how they stand in the marketplace or against their competitors. The SWOT acronym stands for Strengths, Weaknesses, Opportunities, and Threats.

With your partner, analyze yourselves using a SWEAT. Instead of listing opportunities and threats, focus on Strengths, Weaknesses, Excuses, Aspirations, and Targets. Each partner performs an individual SWEAT, and then one together. First, list your own three to five strengths as they relate to your fitness and health goals or your personal fitness journey (e.g., I am great at push-ups; I have strong leg muscles; I am great at staying committed to a training partner). Then list three to five weaknesses (e.g., I have poor posture; my abs are weak; I snack too much in the evenings). Next, list three to five excuses for not achieving your goals (e.g., I get bored after a few weeks of exercises; I get overwhelmed in September when school starts; I have a shoulder injury that I worry about). Then list your three top aspirations. What are your fitness, health or wellness hopes, dreams, and desires? How do you want to feel or look? What do you want to achieve through this process? And lastly, set three targets. These targets should take your excuses into consideration, and create a plan to overcome those roadblocks. Most importantly, your targets are your small and large goals, and your achievement deadline. See appendix B for a SWEAT Self-Worksheet to log your responses.

Once each partner has gone through the process, connect and discuss each point together. By sharing with your workout buddy, you voice your weaknesses or fears, you strengthen your commitment, and you create your goal statement. Accountability is the key to success and putting it out there to a partner or workout buddy boosts the probability for greater success.

additional workout during the week to make up for a shorter one. Progression means that adjustments can be made to the volume of exercise by adjusting any or all three components. For example, as an individual becomes more fit, he may choose to exercise at a higher intensity, add in extra workouts, or work out longer. In general, a gradual progression is preferable, as it may improve exercise adherence and decrease the risk of injuries. However, regularly monitoring of FITT-VP will keep exercise interesting and effective (Deschenes and Garber 2018).

Partner Workout Formats

Designing your partner workouts is dependent on many of the factors discussed earlier in the chapter. Your and your partner's goals, in combination with choosing the fastest and most effective pathway to hit your targets, require planning. As does finding the best training format for you and your partner. Some formats are developed with partners using each other as resistance while others use a more individualized approach. With so many choices, partners can switch from format to format or stick to one before trying something new. Formats to try include the following and are summarized in table 4.2.

Partner Assisted

The partners are both performing two exercises simultaneously, using each other as resistance or support. These exercises are mainly bodyweight focused and slightly more challenging than other formats. For example, one partner holds a high plank and the other performs a push-up on her back. Then they switch roles.

Partner Resisted

The partner adds or acts as the resistance for an exercise. For example, one partner performs a push-up while the other partner exerts pressure on the back to create more resistance.

Partner Equipped

In this format, partners are working with a variety of small equipment. These exercises use different pieces of equipment to enhance a workout performed together. A great example of this is performing abdominal curls while passing a medicine ball to each other.

Partner Cardio

Partner cardio exercises may or may not require equipment. The warm-up could follow a solo format, each partner doing something different, whereas the rest of the workout could incorporate the resistance band. This provides variety and requires some planning and organization.

Partner Solo

Partners are engaged and working out at the same time, but each person is doing a different and separate exercise. This format is ideal for partners that have very different skill sets but still want to exercise together. For example, one partner could do burpees while the other does jumping jacks. Once they complete their reps, they switch. Partner A now does jumping jacks and partner B does burpees.

Table 4.2   Partner and Exercise Format Matchup

	Partner assisted	Partner resisted	Partner equipped	Partner cardio	Partner solo
Evenly matched partner—size, strength, fitness, and effort levels	Yes	Yes	Yes	Yes	Yes
Mismatched partner—size and strength	Modified	Modified	Modified	Yes	Yes
Mismatched partner—fitness and effort levels	Modified	Yes	Modified	Modified	Yes

Coaching Your Partner

Working together with your partner requires that each of you take on the role of personal trainer at some time or another. A personal trainer's purpose is multifaceted. Beyond planning the workout and providing encouraging motivation, a trainer is always looking for ways to correct movement patterns to make certain that each exercise is safe and effective. When training with your workout buddy, it is important to be aware of your own positioning and that of your partner. Always do a quick body scan from head to toe. There are a few common things to watch for, regardless if the exercise is a squat or a push-up, and some simple corrective cues will help both you and your partner on the path to staying injury free. Refer to table 4.3 for posture tips.

Table 4.3   Safe and Effective Posture Tips

Body part	Ideal posture
Head	The head should be in line with the spine. Keep the chin slightly tucked in and the gaze forward.
Shoulders	Draw the shoulder blades back and down. Relax the upper trapezius muscles, creating distance between the shoulders and the ears.
Spine	In neutral spine, lengthen through the back, keep the head in line with the spine, and create an imaginary straight line through the entire body.
Low back	In neutral alignment, there is a slight lumbar curve in the low back. Avoid anything exaggerated (extreme posterior or anterior tilt) unless a movement dictates it.
Upper back	Draw the shoulder blades down and back.
Hips	Whether standing, prone, or in a supine position, the hips should be level.
Knees	Hips, knees, and toes are all in line when standing. When squatting or lunging, avoid the knees going past the toes.
Feet	The feet should be in line with the knees. Generally, feet point forward or there is a slight external rotation of the feet.
Core	Keep the core active and engaged.
Breath	An easy cue to remember, aside from "avoid holding your breath" is to inhale on the preparation of a move, and exhale on the exertion.

Athletic Ready Position

The athletic stance is a common positioning term. It is the foundational basis for athletic development and is fundamental across many activities. The partner exercises in this book often refer to the athletic ready position or athletic stance.

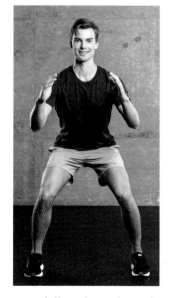

The key to a proper athletic stance is maintaining a neutral spine, hinging slightly forward at the hips, keeping the knees slightly bent, driving the hips back, and keeping the chest lifted. Another key factor is lowering the center of gravity. If you stand too tall or flat footed, you can't move or respond as quickly, or execute a movement pattern with good form. The eyes should be looking forward and not down, and the feet should be approximately shoulder-width apart or slightly wider depending on the individual. Even though an athletic stance is not appropriate for all exercises (e.g., a shoulder press is not executed with a forward lean), it is advantageous for many, especially when there is movement such as in interval drills, agility moves, and plyometrics. Like any exercise progression, a good reminder cue is, "get into position, then move."

PART II

PARTNER EXERCISES

Part II provides partner exercises that focus on bodyweight-training, small-equipment partner-resisted, or cardio-focused exercises. Each exercise begins with a description, followed by the equipment that is needed (if any), movement cues, and a section of teaching tips and variations to make the exercises easier or harder. The challenge level for each partner exercise, based on the complexity of the movements or the physical challenge, is highlighted in a tab on the side of each page.

CHAPTER 5

Bodyweight Exercises

Bodyweight exercises use your body as the resistance. The exercises in this chapter engage both partners simultaneously by performing the same movements or different movements at the same time. It is very important that each partner be aware of their own body positioning as well as that of their partner. Communication is key.

GET-UPS

This exercise focuses on teamwork and coordinated movements. Both partners are engaged but have slightly different roles. It is a full body exercise that will strengthen the legs, upper body, and core, and it includes a pulling movement.

Movement Cues

1. Stand facing each other with the feet wider than hip-width apart in a slightly staggered position and grasp right forearms.
2. Partner A lowers down to sit on the floor while partner B hinges at the hips and continues to hold forearms with partner A.
3. Partner A rolls down onto the back, curls back up, and returns to a standing position without using the left hand to push off the floor.
4. Once standing, the roles reverse and partner B sits, rolls, and stands up.
5. After completing a set, change hand positions and repeat for reps on the other side before partners switch roles.

Tips and Variations

- If either partner has a difficult time standing up without using the opposite hand, the partner must play a more active role in assisting the lift by pulling.
- To increase the challenge, position the feet side by side versus offset, or try to return to standing on one leg rather than both legs.

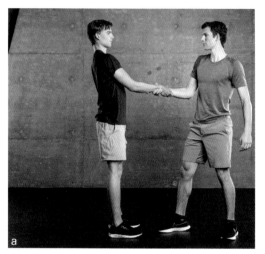

a

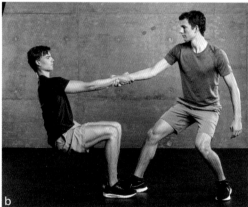

b

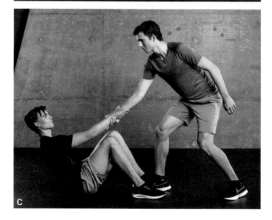

c

PISTOL SQUAT

Single-leg squats are challenging at the best of times. Pistol squats are effective for unilateral training and highlighting muscular imbalances. Performing them with a partner's assistance is the perfect way to train this movement pattern.

Movement Cues

1. Stand facing each other and reach with the right hand to grasp right forearms.
2. The arms should be parallel to the floor, the elbows bent, the shoulders relaxed, and the core active. Partner B's other arm is relaxed along the side or the hand is on the hip.
3. Partner B lifts the left leg straight out in front, flexing the foot.
4. Bend the right leg to lower the glutes toward the floor.
5. Keep the extended left leg straight as it lowers, parallel to the floor, with the hamstring almost touching the floor.
6. Bend or straighten the locked arm to ensure appropriate tension and alignment throughout the exercise.
7. Pause at the bottom, and work together with partner A to straighten the right leg, lifting back up to the start position.
8. Partner B repeats for reps before switching to the other leg.
9. Switch partner roles and repeat for reps.

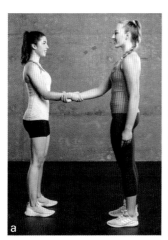 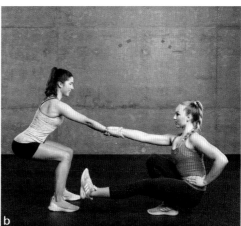

Tips and Variations

- Throughout the movement, try to hold the nonworking leg in the extended position.
- To make the movement easier, avoid squatting as low.
- In its most advanced form, hold the foot of the extended leg with the free arm and repeat the squat motion continuously.

FRONT SQUAT HOLD

This exercise is cooperative and teamwork focused. Partners help each other with the lowering down and lifting portions of the squat. With assistance, a partner can lower into the squat more confidently while holding onto each other with constant pressure through the hands.

Movement Cues

1. Stand facing each other with the feet forward and hip-width apart, the arms raised, and the elbows slightly bent.
2. Lift the hands to shoulder height with the arms extended forward.
3. Partner A reaches for partner B's outstretched hands.
4. With the hands together, partner A slowly lowers toward the floor, pushing the hips behind, into a squat with the assistance of partner B, while maintaining constant and equal pressure.
5. Return to the start position and repeat for reps before switching roles.

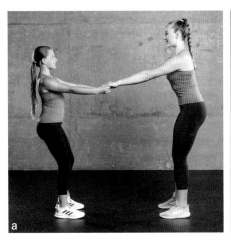 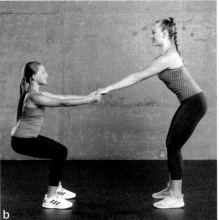

Tips and Variations

- It is important to focus on correct squatting form throughout the entire range of motion.
- If partners are mismatched, the assisting partner may opt for an offset stance for greater stability.
- To increase the challenge, release one set of hands, switching from right- to left-hand holds.

SQUAT AND GLUTE LIFT

Depending on the exercise, occasionally one partner serves as the anchor or holds a stationary position, while the other partner is moving. Regardless of positioning, each partner is still active throughout the exercise and should maintain correct body alignment. In this drill, the lower body gets an intense workout, both while holding a sumo squat and while lifting into a glute bridge.

Movement Cues

1. Facing each other, partner A lies on the floor and partner B stands near partner A's feet.

2. Partner A bends the knees and draws the feet toward the glutes with the heels in line with the sitting bones, keeping the spine and the pelvis in a neutral position.

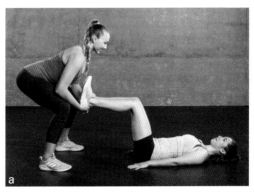

3. The feet should be flat on the floor, the core active, and the arms resting along the sides of the body.

4. Partner B moves closer to partner A's feet and drops down into a wide sumo squat position, keeping the knees behind the ankles and dropping the hips low toward the floor.

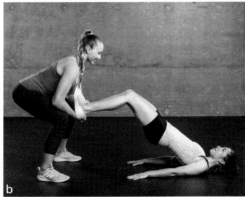

5. Partner B places the forearms on the top of the thighs, shifting the weight slightly back and keeping the spine in a neutral position.

6. Partner A then lifts up both feet and places the heels in partner B's hands; partner B may wish to interlock the fingers.

7. Partner A lengthens through the back, lifts the glutes off

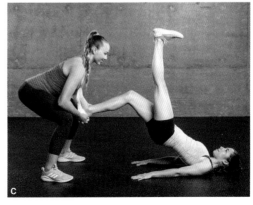

the floor, and moves onto the shoulder blades, keeping the shins parallel to the floor and the knees bent.

8. Partner A lifts one leg and either flexes the foot or points the toes toward the ceiling, lowering and lifting the glutes with the leg extended for reps.

9. Partner B remains in an isometric low squat position for the remainder of the set before the partners switch legs and then switch roles and repeat for reps.

Tips and Variations

- To make the movement easier, omit the leg lift; keep both feet in place, and lift and lower the hips.
- Another less challenging variation is to lightly touch the ground each rep or keep the elevated leg slightly bent versus straight.
- To increase the challenge, partner A lifts and lowers for continuous reps (without touching down) or holds the leg in the air for time versus lifting and lowering.

TABLETOP AND JUMPING JACK

The tabletop position is a fundamental holding move when trying to incorporate exercises against a partner. In the prone tabletop, the knees are on the floor and hands are lined up under the shoulder. This position creates a strong base for partners to work on, over, or alongside each other.

Equipment

- Mat (1; optional)

Movement Cues

1. To begin, partner A starts on the floor in a kneeling, tabletop position on the hands and knees.
2. When in the tabletop, make sure the knees are directly under the hips and the hands are in line with the shoulders.
3. Partner A lifts and extends the left leg, keeping it parallel with the floor.
4. Perpendicular to and on the left side of partner A, partner B places the left hand on partner A's left shoulder and the right hand on partner A's left hip.
5. With light pressure, partner B walks the feet away, keeping the knees slightly bent and in a semiplank position.
6. While maintaining position, partner A stabilizes against the light pressure.
7. Once in position, partner B begins to perform a cardio movement such as jumping jacks, side-to-side hops, or mountain climbers.

8. After the first set is completed, repeat the same move on the other side of the body.

9. Switch partner roles and repeat for reps.

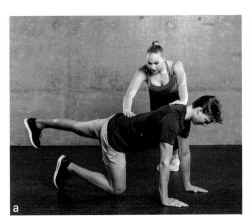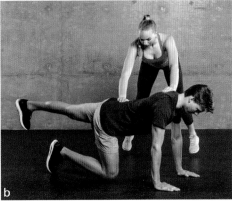

Tips and Variations

• If the partner in the tabletop position needs more stability, both knees can remain on the floor.

• This exercise is more challenging if partners are not similar in size and strength.

REVERSE TABLETOP AND TRICEPS DIP

Reverse tabletop and triceps dip are two exercises that can be executed on their own or performed together in a sequence. As an option, partners may choose to perform these exercises side by side versus on each other.

Movement Cues

1. In this sequence, both partners begin in a standing position, one in front of the other, facing the same direction a couple of feet apart.

2. To begin, partner A sits on the floor with the knees bent and places the hands near the glutes.

3. The hands should be directly under the shoulders, the fingertips together or slightly spread and facing toward the feet.

4. The heels are placed directly in line with the sitting bones and hip-width apart.

5. Partner A lifts the hips up off the floor, maintaining a neutral position with the spine and pelvis, keeping the core engaged, and the neck long.

6. Facing in the same direction, partner B places the hands on partner A's knees and walks the feet forward until the thighs are just above parallel with the floor.

HARD

7. Once in position with the arms straight, knees bent, and feet flat on the floor, partner B bends and straightens the elbows to execute a triceps dip.

8. Partner A holds the reverse tabletop while partner B completes the triceps dip repetitions.

9. Switch partner roles and repeat for reps.

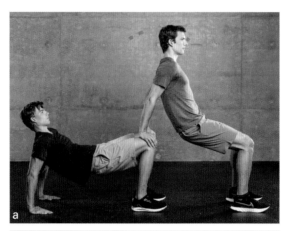

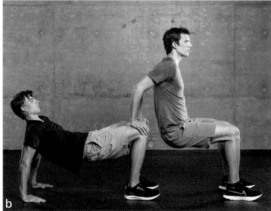

Tips and Variations

- It is important to keep the feet, knees, and hands on the knees aligned, and the shoulders in line with the elbows and wrists throughout both exercises.

- If the straight arm reverse tabletop is too challenging to hold, opt for a bridge position, with the shoulders on the floor and the hips lifted into a bridge position.

- To increase the challenge, partners can alternate exercises. Partner A does a triceps dip and holds while partner B drops the glutes to the floor and then lifts back into the reverse tabletop. Repeat.

PLANK AND ROW

Finding effective pulling movement patterns with bodyweight training can be a challenge. This exercise uses your partner's bodyweight as resistance to work the back of the body.

Equipment
- Mat (1; optional)

Movement Cues
1. To begin, partner A places the hands on the floor, elbows under the shoulders, and walks the legs back until they are extended, feet positioned slightly wider than hip-width apart and the toes tucked under, then lifting up into a high straight-arm plank position. Shoulder blades are together, and the chest is open.
2. Partner A keeps the core very active and the torso in a neutral position.
3. Partner B stands with a slight knee bend and neutral spine in between Partner A's feet, then hinges from the hip to pick up each of partner A's legs, holding them just above the ankles.
4. Partner B slightly bends the knees, lowering partner A's legs until they are parallel with the floor.
5. While in this squat position, partner B begins to row partner A's legs slowly and with control; moving them from a low to high position, while contracting through the back muscles and keeping the eyes slightly forward.
6. Partner A focuses on keeping the body position long and strong.
7. Once the reps are completed, partner B lowers partner A's feet back to the floor and partners switch positions to repeat for reps.

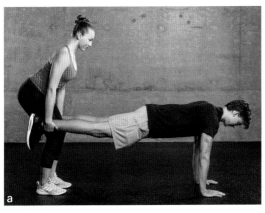 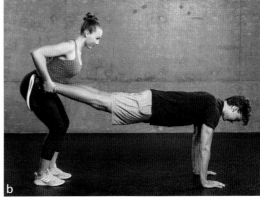

Tips and Variations
- Correct body position by both partners is extremely important.
- When performing the rowing action, move slowly and with control. This exercise should never be performed quickly.

WHEELBARROW PUSH-UP AND SQUAT

Similar to the upcoming plank and row exercise, this drill is a combination of two moves. It also requires lifting and proper body control by both participants. A prerequisite for the exercise is the ability to hold a full body high plank position. Take time to get into and out of the exercise.

Equipment

- Mat (1; optional)

Movement Cues

1. To begin, partner A starts on the floor in a kneeling, tabletop position on the hands and knees. The hands are under the shoulders, the core is active, and the shoulders are stabilized.

2. Partner A moves into a plank by extending the legs back, tucking the toes under, while keeping the arms straight with the shoulder blades together and chest open, and maintains neutral alignment through the torso, hips level, and legs straight.

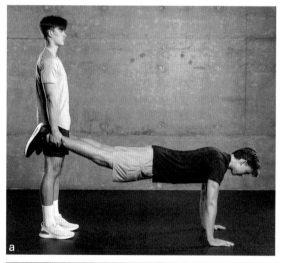

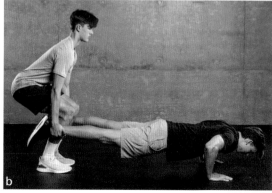

3. Partner B squats down to grasp both of partner A's legs at the ankles and holds them at approximately midthigh height, with partner A's feet approximately hip-width apart.

4. Partner A adjusts the arm position and performs a push-up, lowering the chest toward the floor, then pressing the hands into the floor to return to the high plank position.

5. As partner A lowers into the push-up, partner B squats down, shifting the weight back, keeping the chest lifted, and driving through the feet to lift back up as both partners return to the starting position.

6. Repeat for reps before switching roles.

7. To switch positions, lower partner A's feet to the floor one at a time.

Tips and Variations

- Avoid spending too much time in the high plank position if either partner has wrist issues.

- To make the movements easier, partners can alternate the exercises: partner A performs a push-up, then partner B performs a squat, rather than doing the exercises at the same time.

- As an additional exercise option, try the wheelbarrow walk: while partner B holds the legs, partner A walks the hands forward one step at a time.

WALK OUT AND CLAP

Partners move simultaneously in this full body exercise. Once the ideal distance from each other is determined and the correct movement pattern is achieved, the goal is to increase the tempo of the exercise while maintaining good body control.

Movement Cues

1. Stand facing each other, a little more than a full body-length apart.

2. Each partner lowers the hands slowly to the floor, hinging from the hips with straight legs, and moving the crown of the head toward the floor with the chin tucked in.

3. Once the hands reach the floor, walk the hands forward into a plank position.

4. Partners clap right hands together, then left hands together, before walking the hands back in toward the feet and standing up.

5. Repeat for reps.

MODERATE

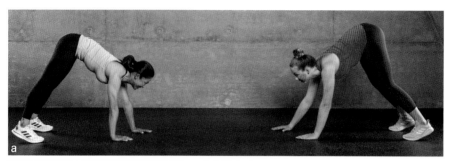

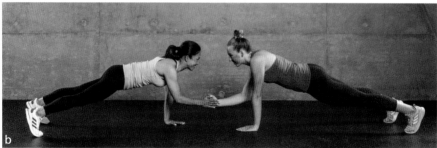

Tips and Variations

- To increase the challenge, pick up the pace of the exercise or reach the hands over the head in the standing position.
- To further increase the challenge, add an extra set of claps to each repetition. For example, on the first repetition, clap right and left hands once; second set, two sets of claps; third set, three sets of claps; and so on, holding the plank longer each time as you add hand claps.

DOWN DOG CRAWL

This fun drill combines two very different moves: one partner holds a stationary position and the other partner is running and crawling. Because the floor surface makes a difference when crawling, opt for a softer surface or use a couple of mats.

Equipment

- Mat (1; optional)

Movement Cues

1. To begin, partner A starts in a straight-arm plank position by extending the legs back and tucking the toes under, maintaining neutral alignment through the torso and hips level. Shoulder blades are together, and the chest is open.

MODERATE

2. From the plank, partner A walks the hands back toward the feet, lifting the hips up into a pike position. In yoga, this position is called the Downward Facing Dog. The arms and legs are straight, the head is in line with the spine, and the core is active. Partner A holds that position.

3. Partner B starts in a standing position on the outside of partner A's left hand.

4. Partner B lowers to the floor and quickly crawls under partner A, ending up near partner A's right foot.

5. Once through, partner B stands up and runs around to partner A's left foot, lowers to the floor and crawls under partner A again, ending up near partner A's right hand.

6. Repeat the figure-eight run and crawl movements in both directions before switching roles.

7. Complete a minimum of two sets in each direction.

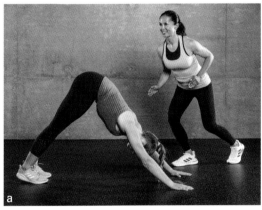

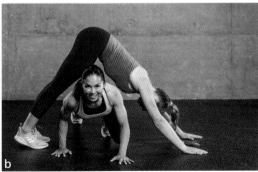

Tips and Variations

- The higher partner A's hips are in the pike position, the easier it is for partner B to crawl under and around.

- To increase the challenge, accelerate the tempo of the crawl, stand, and run.

CRAB AND REACH

This floor-based exercise is a combined version of the crab dip and the crab walk from years past. Both partners are on the floor for this total body exercise that works the shoulders, upper back, triceps, lower body, and core.

Movement Cues

1. To begin, partners sit side by side on the floor about two feet apart, facing the same direction.
2. Both partners lift up into a reverse tabletop. Hands are under the shoulders with finger tips toward the glutes, and the feet forward.
3. Partners simultaneously bend the elbows dropping slightly into a triceps dip.
4. Both partners lift their outside hands off the floor, extend their arms, and reach up and over, bringing the palms of their hands together.
5. Return the hands to the start position and repeat for reps before switching sides.

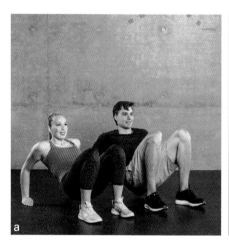 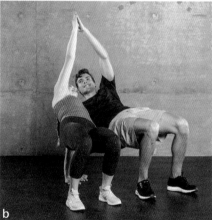

Tips and Variations

- To make the movement easier, position closer together and eliminate the triceps dip.
- To increase the challenge, try to reach farther and increase the tempo of the exercise.

SNOWBOARDER

If you have ever been snowboarding and remember your first day on the mountain, you will appreciate this exercise. Chances are, you spent just as much time sitting on the snow as you did standing on your board. In this movement, partners transition from floor to standing as quickly as possible.

Movement Cues

1. Stand back-to-back.
2. Stepping laterally approximately three feet away from each other, partners transition to a seated position on the floor with the arms at the sides and close to the glutes, fingertips pointing toward the feet, the knees slightly bent and the feet flat on the floor.
3. Both partners straighten the arms, lifting the glutes off the floor, and move into a semireverse tabletop position.

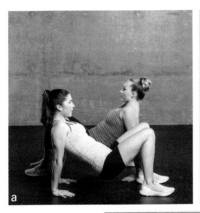
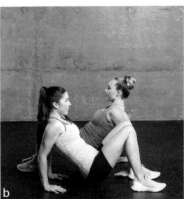
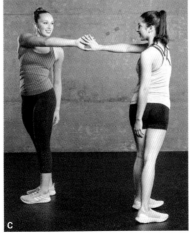

4. Both partners perform a triceps dip by bending the elbows, dropping the glutes toward the floor, then straightening the arms to lift the glutes back up.

5. Partners perform two to three triceps dips simultaneously.

6. To return to standing, shift the body weight slightly to the right, and use the right arm to press into the floor and stand.

7. Once standing, partners rotate to high five with the right hand before turning back around and quickly lowering again to the floor.

8. Repeat continuously, trying to increase the speed of triceps dips and high fives before switching hands and repeating reps on the left.

Tips and Variations

- Be aware of wrist positioning, and make sure each partner is comfortable with the movements.
- Coordinating the timing with your partner is tricky; start slowly to learn the movement pattern first.
- Getting up off the floor into a stand is the hardest part of the exercise, especially on the nondominant side; modify as needed.
- To increase the challenge, accelerate the tempo of the exercise.

SURFER POP-UP

If you ever watch surfers, it is amazing to see how quickly they transition from lying down on their boards to standing up, in one fluid motion. The movement takes an incredible amount of strength and balance. Training on land is an opportunity to practice the skills that will build lower body, upper body, and core strength—a true full body conditioning exercise.

Movement Cues

1. Lie prone on the floor, head to head, and approximately one to two feet away from each other.

2. The elbows are bent at the sides and tucked in, palms of the hands on the floor, and feet relaxed.

3. Slide the hands down toward the armpits and tuck the toes under.

4. Transition into a low plank, lifting the body off the floor.

5. Next, jump the feet in toward the shoulders while at the same time, lifting the hands off the floor, landing in a low crouch position.

6. Partners give each other an "air" high 10 in the low squat position before placing the hands back on the floor, walking out the feet, and lowering to the floor into a plank position again.

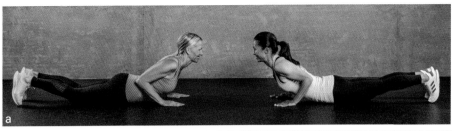

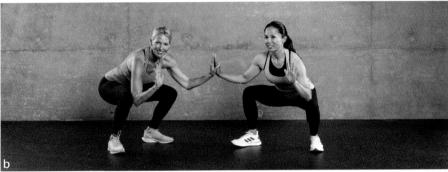

7. Repeat the sequencing from step 5 with the option to add a slight rotation, turning and angling slightly away from each other, and connecting with a high five instead of a high 10 (because of the rotation).

8. Repeat for reps.

Tips and Variations

- Because the movement requires a great deal of power to jump the feet in and lift the hands up off the floor at the same time, separating the motions will help: Lift into a plank first, next hop in the feet while staying low, and finish by lifting the hands.

- To increase the challenge, speed up the movements.

KNEELING PUSH-UP WITH ROTATION

When learning to do a proper push-up, start with the basics. A kneeling push-up is a good alternative to its full-body counterpart. If partners have different abilities, this drill works well with any type of push-up.

Movement Cues

1. Partners begin side by side, each in a tabletop position on all fours.

2. Partners walk the hands out until both are in a kneeling plank position, hands slightly wider than shoulder-width apart. Shoulder blades are together and the chest is open.

3. Both partners lower the chest to the floor, allowing the elbows to bend and extend outward.

EASY

4. Press down into the hands to return to the start position, then both partners lift the outside hand off the floor and reach in front to clap hands with their partner.
5. Bring the hands back to the floor and perform the next push-up, repeating the pattern.
6. Once the set is complete, switch sides and repeat the set.

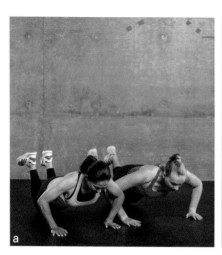 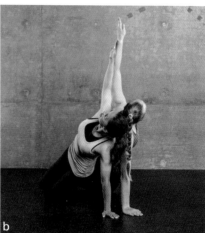

Tips and Variations

*   To increase the challenge, perform the exercise in a full push-up position, or attempt to lift the inside leg as you rotate the opposite hand in front to clap.
*   Lower the body to a depth in which you can hold proper alignment.

PLANK AND PUSH-UP

Combining two classic exercises in one drill is a perfect way to get more done in less time. Decrease the difficulty by modifying the position or movements if necessary. It is important in these challenging exercises to communicate well with each other.

Equipment

*   Mat (1; optional)

Movement Cues

1. In this drill, partners perform separate exercises while in contact with each other.

HARD

2. Partner A starts on the floor, kneeling in tabletop position with the hands under the shoulders, the core active, and the shoulders stabilized.

3. Partner A extends the legs back, tucking the toes under, to come into a high straight-arm plank position, maintaining neutral alignment through the torso and hips level. The shoulder blades are together, and the chest is open.

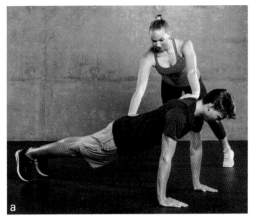

4. Standing perpendicular to and on the left side of partner A, partner B places the left hand on partner A's left shoulder blade and the right hand on Partner A's left hip.

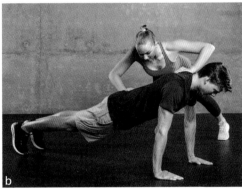

5. Partner B walks the feet back into a plank position and then performs an incline push-up.

6. During the push-up, partner B should keep the spine neutral, the core active, the hips and the head in line with the spine, the hands wide, and the elbows bent.

7. Partner B performs all repetitions on partner A's left side, then repeats on partner A's right side. Both partners rest and then switch roles and repeat for reps.

Tips and Variations

- To make the move easier, switch out the straight-arm plank for a forearm plank and the full body push-up for a kneeling push-up.

- To decrease the challenge, modify the push-up by keeping the knees bent and the feet positioned closer toward your partner; this will take some of the weight off the partner's back.

- Always place the hands on the partner's bony parts of the body (i.e., shoulder blade, hip bone, etc.).

HANDSTAND

If you are working toward executing and mastering a handstand, this exercise is an ideal precursor to that popular yoga pose. This move requires a great deal of overall strength, core stability, upper body movement, and confidence in your partner.

Movement Cues

1. Partner A starts in a tabletop position on all fours with the hands under the shoulders, the core active, the shoulders stabilized. Partner A then extends the legs back, tucking the toes under, to come into a high straight-arm plank position, maintaining neutral alignment through the torso and hips level. The shoulder blades are together, and the chest is open.

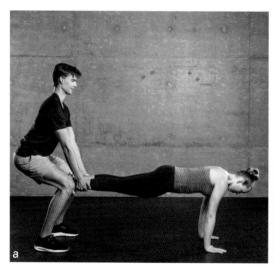
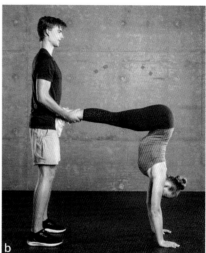
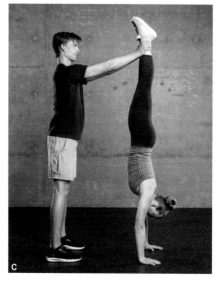

2. Partner B places a hand on each of partner A's ankles to hold the feet.

3. Partner A begins to walk the hands in toward the feet, while partner B adjusts the hold on partner A's ankles as needed.

4. Partner A can stop when in a pike position with the legs level and parallel to partner B's waist, and the torso is in a vertical position.

5. For partner A to move into a handstand, partner B must switch hand positions from an overhand to an underhand grip, and adjust the hands under each shin.

6. Partner A returns to walking in the hands as partner B then lifts partner A's feet straight up into the air, into a straight handstand.

7. Partner B lowers partner A's legs back down toward the floor and switch roles and repeat for reps.

Tips and Variations

- Good communication between partners is important to execute the exercise correctly.
- Avoid performing a handstand immediately after any cardio work.

STRAIGHT-LEG LIFT

Working the abdominals with the legs straight and lifted instead of with the knees bent and feet on the floor is a challenging way to mix up an ab routine. It is important that the movements are done with control and that each partner is physically able to execute the movements with proper technique.

MODERATE

Equipment

- Mat (1; optional)

Movement Cues

1. Partner A lies faceup on the floor, and partner B stands just behind partner A's head.

2. Partner A reaches back and holds onto both of partner B's lower legs, while partner B extends the arms, so they are parallel to the floor.

3. While maintaining good positioning, partner A lifts the legs straight up to the ceiling, contracting the abs and keeping the back in a neutral position.

4. Partner A lifts the feet toward partner B's extended arms to tap the feet to partner B's hands.

5. Partner B may choose to give partner A's legs a light push, causing partner A to respond by resisting with control before lowering the legs slowly back down to the floor.

6. Another option could involve partner B holding out a target with the hands six inches higher than partner A's extended leg.

7. Partner A lifts the glutes up off the floor and attempts to tap the target with the toes, before lowering the glutes down and repeating. Adjust the target as needed.

8. Repeat for reps before switching partners.

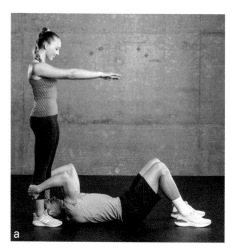 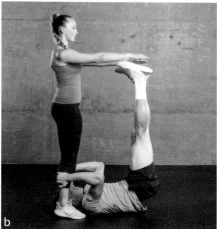

Tips and Variations

- To do this exercise properly, partners must be able to maintain proper low back positioning and avoid arching through the back.
- To make the movement easier, only lower the legs to the height in which you can maintain proper back positioning.

CURL-UP AND GIVE ME 10

Working the core and abs is an exercise foundation and a favorite. In this drill, you and your partner work in tandem on the same move but reach in the middle to connect with a two-handed high 10.

Equipment

- Mats (2; optional)

Movement Cues

1. Both partners sit facing each other with the knees bent and the feet on the floor.

2. The ankles should be slightly overlapping.

3. To begin, both partners roll back, contracting the abdominals, and keeping the rib cage down. The chin should be slightly tucked into the chest.

4. Focus on lowering and curling through the spine one vertebra at a time, until the low back touches the floor.

5. Partners then roll up at the same time, maintaining a gentle curve in the spine and finishing in a tall seated position, giving each other a high 10.

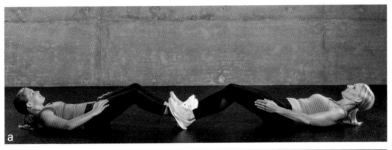

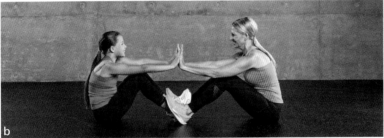

Tips and Variations

- To make the curls easier, position the hands at the sides of the legs or hold onto the legs for assistance.
- To increase the challenge, extend the arms overhead in the start position and keep them extended as you curl up.

BICYCLE CRUNCH

Bicycle crunches are a great exercise to fire up the rectus abdominis muscles and the obliques. With bicycles, faster isn't always better. Focus on slow, controlled movements.

Equipment

- Mats (2; optional)

Movement Cues

1. Partners lie on their backs, feet to feet, with the elbows bent and the hands behind the head.

2. Positioning is important; adjustments may need to be made based on leg lengths, as both partners need to extend one leg at a time.

MODERATE

3. Partners press the bottoms of the feet together, keeping the shins parallel to the floor, maintaining resistance through the feet.

4. By communicating with your partner, decide who will start the movement.

5. Partner A begins by pressing slightly harder and extending the right leg while partner B bends the left knee; then the bicycle movement begins with the legs bending and straightening in a coordinated fashion.

6. At the same time, lift the head slightly off the floor and rotate to bring the elbow to the opposite knee that is closer to the head. Continue to complete these movements alternating the opposite elbow to the opposite knee each time.

7. Repeat for reps.

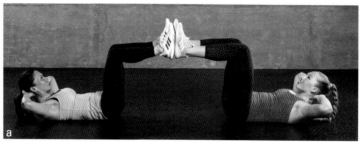

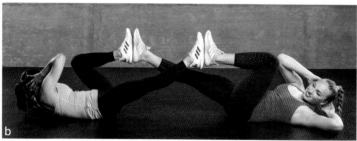

Tips and Variations

- Both partners should try to keep even pressure through the feet.
- To add variety, change the tempo; start at a steady pace then slow it down or add 1-2 second holds every few rotations.

MODERATE

V-SIT CIRCLE

V-sits challenge the core and require good alignment. If sitting in a V-position is uncomfortable, make adjustments by sitting up higher versus leaning back, or modify by placing one foot on the floor.

Equipment

- Mats (2; optional)

Movement Cues

1. Partners sit on the floor facing each other, feet on the floor, knees slightly bent and hands grasping behind the thighs or resting on the floor.
2. Both partners lean slightly back, keeping the spine in a neutral position and forming a V-shape with the torso and legs.
3. Both partners lift their feet off the floor, shins parallel to the floor and feet close.
4. Partner B starts by holding the legs in a stationary position while partner A rotates their legs around partner B's legs in one full clockwise rotation, and then switches and rotates the legs in one full counterclockwise rotation.
5. Partners switch roles so that partner A's legs are stationary while partner B's legs rotate.
6. Continue, repeating the back-and-forth circular movements clockwise and counterclockwise for reps.

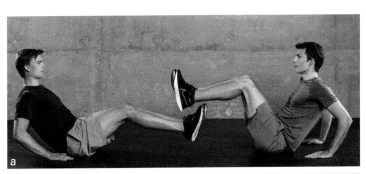

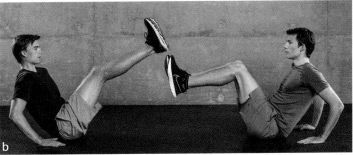

Tips and Variations

- Avoid flexing through the spine or letting the hips roll back.
- As an option, partner A and partner B simultaneously circle the feet.
- To increase the challenge, lift the legs higher or lift the hands off the floor.

HARD

UP-AND-OVER ABS

In this active abdominal exercise, partners can use the sequence as a tempo drill and even compete against other partner groups to see who can complete the most reps within a set amount of time.

Equipment

- Mats (2; optional)

Movement Cues

1. Partners lie faceup on the floor with their right shoulders next to each other, knees bent, and the feet flat on the floor.
2. Partner A slides the right arm under partner B's bent legs and grasps partner's B's left hand; partner B does the same thing and grasps the opposite hands; arms remain on the floor.
3. While holding hands, both partners draw their knees in and lift their legs straight up to the ceiling.
4. Once the legs are extended, both partners lift the hips up, pressing the upper back into the floor, lengthening through the legs and pressing the feet straight up to the ceiling.
5. Next, simultaneously, partners sweep the legs up and over, shifting the hips, and then lowering the legs toward the floor into a pike position.
6. Return the legs back up and over so that the feet are toward the ceiling again; reposition the left hips together and rest the low back once again on the floor.
7. Repeat in a continuous up-and-over motion for reps.

Tips and Variations

- To increase the challenge, accelerate the pace of the movement while maintaining the correct body positions.
- Challenge other partner pairings to see who can complete the most reps in a set amount of time.

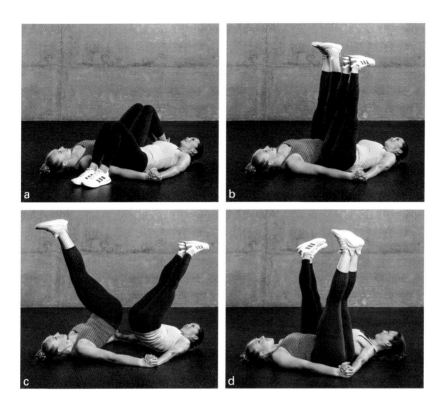

BACK EXTENSION

Most tasks in our daily lives happen in front of our bodies. Whether it is walking, texting, lifting children, or driving, we live in a face-first world. Our movement patterns tend to include a great deal of forward flexion. To keep ourselves standing tall and our backs strong and not overstretched, extension work is a great equalizer.

Equipment

- Mats (2; optional)

Movement Cues

1. Both partners lie prone on the floor, feet to feet, with the hands resting under the forehead.
2. Partners hook their feet around each other; one partner keeps the legs to the inside, and the other partner wraps the feet around the outside of the other partner's feet.
3. At the same time, both partners pull the belly button up and toward the spine, extending through the spine and upper back, and lifting the chest off the floor.

EASY

4. The arms lift off the floor as the upper body lifts.
5. Feet press into each other while keeping the abdominals engaged to support the back.
6. Hold at the top of the extension for a few breaths before lowering down and repeating the movement for reps.

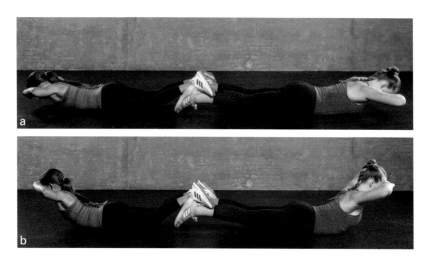

Tips and Variations

- To make the movement easier, avoid lifting and extending too high.
- To simplify the move even more, place the forearms on the floor to assist with the lift and support the extension.
- To increase the challenge, extend the arms long to create length and lift throughout the body.

CHAPTER 6

Partner-Resisted Exercises

Partner-resisted exercises are also body weight focused but with the addition of your partner adding more variable resistance to a movement to make it more challenging. The partner presses on a body part temporarily adding pressure or in some cases at a specific point in the movement pattern. Great care should be taken to ensure the correct amount of resistance is provided. Too little resistance won't provide enough challenge in the exercise, and too much resistance may make your partner incapable of completing the reps and could potentially cause injury. Once again, proper communication between partners is very important. To better understand the concept of adding resistance, bring both your palms together in a prayer position and push the hands together as hard as possible. The resistance felt is called an isometric contraction. The muscles needed to push the hands together are activated, but they are not lengthening (eccentric muscle contraction) or shortening (concentric muscular contraction). Next, push the palms against each other again, but push the right hand harder than the left, shifting the elbow to the left. Return to center. Repeat to the right, moving across the body. Just enough resistance in either direction adds some challenge, but still allows movement. Allowing movement with resistance is the goal of many of the exercises.

WALL SIT

No wall? No problem when you have a partner. The muscles are engaged during the isometric contraction in the holding squat, but there is no movement. Once holding the position, the lower body muscles work hard to keep the rest of the body in position.

Movement Cues

1. Stand back-to-back and link arms.
2. Using moderate pressure to begin, press the backs into each other.
3. Working together, slowly walk out the feet, increasing and maintaining the upper body counterpressure against your partner.
4. Bend the knees to lower the hips into a squat position until the thighs are parallel to the floor.
5. Hold the position for time, focusing on pressing against each other through the back, keeping the hips stable and the core active.
6. Repeat for reps.

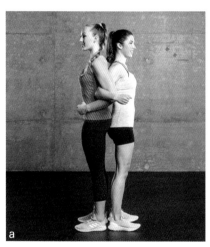 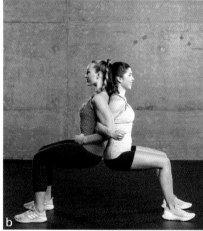

Tips and Variations

- To modify the movement, don't squat as low or hold as long.
- To increase the challenge, perform an upper body movement such as a shoulder press with a weight while staying in a low squat position.
- To further increase the challenge, lift one leg off the floor and hold.

BACK-TO-BACK WALKOUT

Linking arms and lowering each other to the floor simultaneously is a movement that initially seems intimidating but has a fast learning curve. This fun and trust-building exercise encourages partners to communicate. By talking with each other, partners can quickly master the steps.

Movement Cues

1. Stand back-to-back and link arms.

2. Press backs into each other.

3. Working together, lower to the floor by slowly walking the feet away from each other while maintaining upper body counterpressure against your partner.

4. Once seated on the floor with the legs extended, bend the knees and walk the feet back in, gradually returning to a standing position.

5. As the skill improves, you will be able to get up faster just by pushing off the floor with the legs.

6. Repeat for reps.

Tips and Variations

- This drill has a similar degree of difficulty when partners are of matching sizes and strengths.

- This exercise is more challenging if partners are not similar in size and strength.

- To increase the challenge, accelerate the tempo of the lifting and lowering phases.

- Another challenge option is to perform the lifting portion of the exercise using only one leg: Both partners lift their left leg, and rise up using only the right leg. Switch legs on the next lift.

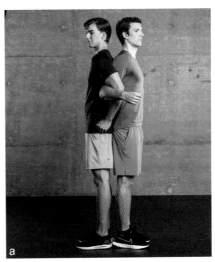

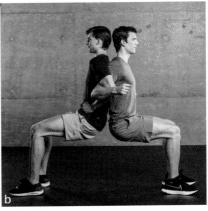

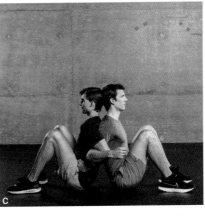

HARD

PUSHOVER PRESS

This exercise is a good icebreaker, especially for partners who are new to working out together. It is very difficult to push your partner off balance, which is not the true intent of this exercise. This exercise is meant to focus on core activation, upper body strength, and lower body stability versus movement. It is also an effective exercise for teaching the benefits of core activation and how a strong core is beneficial with stability and strength in all movements.

Movement Cues

1. Stand facing each other, approximately one to two feet apart.
2. Step forward with the right foot into an offset stance.
3. Lift the hands to approximately shoulder height, positioning them palm to palm with the partner.
4. Lower into an athletic ready position, knees slightly bent, center of gravity low, and core active.
5. On the count of three, both partners push as hard as they can against each other without moving the feet, with the goal of trying to push each other off balance.
6. Partners push for approximately 5 to 10 seconds; rest and repeat with the left foot forward.
7. Repeat for reps.

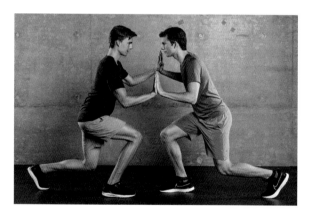

Tips and Variations

- During the pushing phase, partners should automatically drop into a deeper athletic position.
- As an option, a ball (e.g., stability ball) can be used as a partner go-between and an alternative to pressing the palms together.

LUNGE AND PRESS

The lunge and press partner exercise improves core conditioning, lower body strength, and balance. It is also an excellent exercise for connecting with your partner in a fun and challenging way. This exercise is another good icebreaker for new partners.

Movement Cues

1. Stand facing each other, approximately two feet apart.
2. Step forward with the right foot, and lower into a lunge position with the right foot approximately one foot away from the partner's right foot.
3. With right arms lifted and elbows bent, press the right hands together to add some light pressure.
4. While in the lunge position, bend the front leg at the knee to slowly lower down toward the floor and then straighten the leg to come back to the top of the lunge.

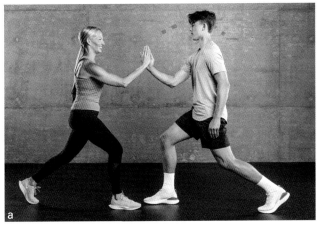

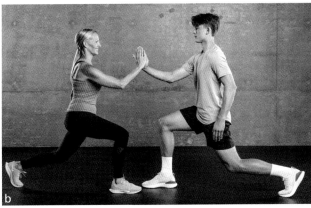

5. Increase the amount of pressure through the right hands during the lowering and lifting.

6. Repeat for reps before switching feet and hand positions.

Tips and Variations

- If the exercise is too challenging, try a squat. Face the opposite direction, two feet apart, with the arm lifted, and right hands connected, lowering and lifting in a squat position. Repeat for reps then switch directions and hand positions.

- To increase the challenge of the base move, place the left hands together above the right hands, adding pressure. Begin lowering in the lunge position then cooperatively release the right hands, keeping the left hands together, as you start to lift. Continue lowering and lifting in the lunge position with the left hands together.

LEG PRESS

Who needs an expensive leg press machine when you have a partner? This do-it-yourself exercise effectively works the lower body muscles and the core, and provides options to make the exercise simpler or ultrachallenging!

Equipment

- Mats (2; optional)

Movement Cues

1. Partners lie on their backs on the floor facing each other. The knees are bent with the feet drawn toward the glutes, and partner A's knees are in line with partner B's knees.

2. The feet should be flat on the floor, the core active, and the arms resting along the sides of the body.

3. Next, partners press the soles of their right feet together, knees bent, and the shins parallel to the floor.

4. Before any movement, press the feet together to create an isometric contraction, or equal pressure between partners A and B.

5. When ready, partner A presses slightly harder and straightens the right leg while partner B slightly resists and bends the right knee (a).

6. Then reverse: Partner B straightens the right leg and partner A bends the right knee.

7. The back-and-forth seesawing movement continues, with partners communicating about the correct amount of pressure to apply.

8. Complete the sets, then repeat with the opposite leg (press left feet together) for reps.

HARD

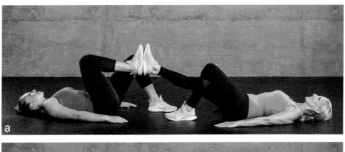

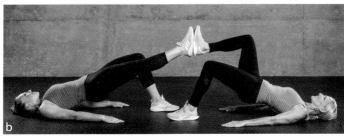

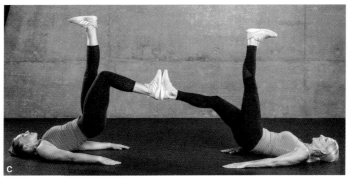

Tips and Variations

- Finding the correct pressure (equal and steady) through the feet, and communicating well with your partner is the key to success for this exercise.

- To increase the challenge, partners can put their feet together, place the hands to the sides, and lift the hips into a shoulder bridge position while performing the movement *(b)*.

- For the ultimate challenge, stay in the shoulder bridge and both partners lift the left legs off of the floor as well. Perform the press while keeping consistent pressure on the right feet and control throughout the body *(c)*.

EASY

RESISTED HAMSTRING CURL

In this exercise, one partner lies prone on the floor, with one knee bent, and the heel lifted, while the other partner adds resistance to the curl-in motion. The key to success in this exercise is creating and maintaining an isometric contraction before adding movement. The term *isometric* refers to muscles that are activated without movement. Once movement begins, the muscles lengthen and shorten with the resistance coming from an outside source: a partner.

Equipment

- Mat (1; optional)

Movement Cues

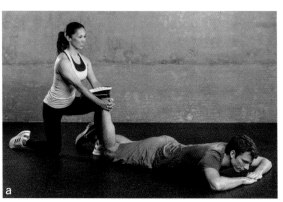

1. Partner A lies prone on the floor, the elbows to the side, and the head slightly lifted or resting on the back of crossed-over hands.

2. Partner B kneels at partner A's feet.

3. Partner A bends the right knee, the thigh on the floor, keeping the opposite leg straight, bringing the foot toward the glutes.

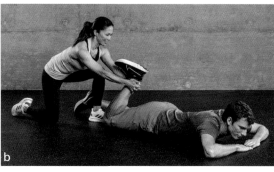

4. Partner B clasps partner A's right ankle. Partner A then tries to draw the heel toward the glutes while partner B creates just enough resistance to make it challenging.

5. Partner A then begins to straighten the leg, returning to the start position as partner B continues to add resistance.

6. Repeat for reps, switch legs, and then reverse roles.

Tips and Variations

- Avoid applying too much resistance; offer enough resistance in both the concentric and eccentric motions to allow movement.

- It is important to communicate in this exercise to find the correct level of resistance.

- Each partner should maintain proper body positioning in their respective roles.

- Avoid arching through the back or twisting during the in-and-out motion of the hamstring curl.

GLUTE BRIDGE LIFT

The glute bridge is not only a challenging exercise for the hamstrings, glutes, lower back, core, and abs, but also very effective with both partners taking an active role in the exercise. Working well together is the key to the success of this partner exercise.

Equipment

- Mats (2; optional)

Movement Cues

1. Partners lie on their backs, toe to toe, the knees bent and the feet very close to the glutes, with the arms at the sides, palms down, and the head on the floor.
2. Partners press the bottoms of their feet together, activating the glutes and lifting the hips off the floor.
3. Lift the feet up as high as possible until the shins are parallel to the floor, maintaining resistance through the feet, and holding in the bridge position for two to four seconds.
4. Simultaneously lower the hips toward the floor while engaging the core, the glutes, and the hamstrings.
5. Repeat for reps.

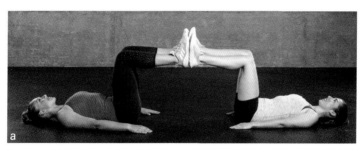

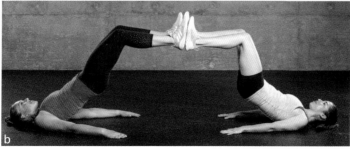

Tips and Variations

- Keep the arms on the floor for balance and control.
- To decrease the challenge, avoid lifting the hips as high and touch the low back down between reps.
- To increase the challenge, lift the arms straight up to the ceiling while performing the lower body movement.

GLUTE BRIDGE BICYCLE

There are many ways partners can add variation and challenge to a double bridge exercise. In this recumbent bike-style move, partners lift up into a bridge position and add a bicycling movement by alternating the pressing action of the legs.

Equipment

- Mats (2; optional)

Movement Cues

1. Partners lie on their backs, toe to toe, the knees bent, and the feet very close to the glutes, with the arms at the sides and the head on the floor.

2. Partners press the bottoms of their feet together and lift the hips off the floor until the shins are parallel to the floor, maintaining resistance through the feet.

3. Holding the bridge position, partner A extends the right leg while partner B bends the left knee. Partner B extends the left leg while partner A bends the right knee. Partners alternate the pushing motion to bicycle the legs back and forth.

4. Repeat for reps or time.

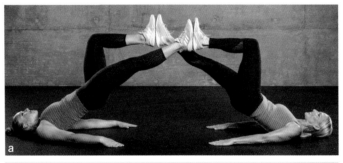

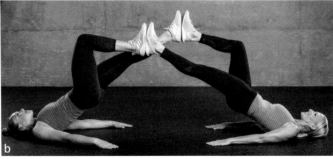

Tips and Variations

- Press the arms into the floor for balance and control.
- Work together to create a smooth bicycle motion.
- To make the movement easier, keep the low back on the floor and alternate the legs.
- To increase the challenge, lift the feet higher and increase the tempo.

RESISTED FRONT AND SIDE RAISE

A front raise is an isolation exercise targeting the front of the shoulders (the anterior deltoids) and a number of secondary muscles, such as the trapezius and pectoralis. The side raise targets the lateral deltoid muscles, located on the sides of the shoulder. The exercise is typically performed with dumbbells, but in this version, your workout partner provides the resistance. Communication is key in both the lifting and lowering of the arms in either the front or side positions.

Movement Cues

1. For the front raise, stand facing each other.
2. Partner A extends the arms in front of the body, just slightly off the thighs.
3. Partner B places the hands against partner A's forearms.
4. Partner A begins to slowly raise the arms, lifting no higher than shoulder height. Partner B offers resistance during the entire movement, both during the lifting and lowering of the arms *(a)*.
5. For the side lateral raises, Partner A lifts the arms out to the side.
6. Partner B stands in front and again offers resistance on both the lifting and lowering *(b)*.
7. Repeat for reps before switching positions.

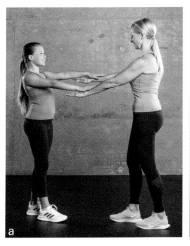
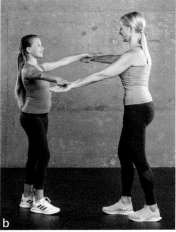

Tips and Variations

- Partners should avoid adding too much resistance. The goal is to be able to lift and lower the arms.
- To decrease the risk of shoulder impingement, slightly turn the thumbs up at the top of the movement and avoid lifting the arms above shoulder height.
- For stronger positioning, ensure the core is active throughout the entire movement.

RESISTED TABLETOP

The tabletop position is an excellent exercise that addresses both stability and mobility, especially in the two-point position in which one leg and the opposite arm are extended. When executing the exercise, concentrate on keeping the muscles of the core actively engaged and lengthening through the spine.

Equipment

- Mats (2; optional)

Movement Cues

1. Partners start in tabletop position facing each other, approximately one to two feet apart, hands and knees on the floor.
2. Place the hands directly under the shoulders and knees directly under the hips, creating a straight line from the hip to the knee.
3. Spread the fingertips wide and stabilize the shoulder girdle.
4. Contract the core muscles, maintaining a neutral spine.
5. At the same time, both partners lift and extend their left legs.
6. Maintaining the neutral spine alignment and not dropping through the hips on the opposite side, extend the right arm straight out and place the right palms against each other.
7. Press the palms of the hands together to create resistance. Offer more resistance as you hold the position.
8. Hold for time, lower the leg, then lower the arm, and switch to the other side and repeat for reps.

EASY

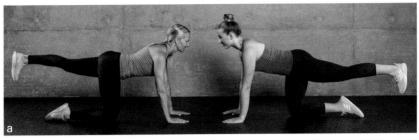

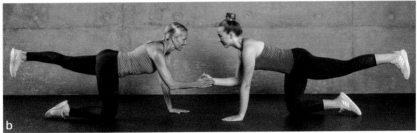

Tips and Variations

- Try to maintain a straight line from the extended arm all the way through to the extended leg.
- To make the movement easier, start with the knees wider and don't lift the leg; use only the arms.
- To increase the challenge, add movement to the extended leg. Draw the lifted leg out to the side of the body in a controlled fashion, then return to the start, or pull the knee into the chest and then straighten the leg, while keeping pressure through the arms.

RESISTED PUSH-UP

Push-ups are simple to make easier or more challenging. Whether it's performing the push-up in a standing position and pressing against the wall, in a tabletop version on all fours, or in a kneeling position, there are many ways to make this classic move easier. Similarly, adding challenging partner progressions is straightforward as well. Mastering the full body push-up can morph into other advanced versions such as a triceps push-up, a tripod position, or a resisted version as described here.

EASY

Equipment

- Mat (1; optional)

Movement Cues

1. Partner A starts in a tabletop position with the hands under the shoulders, the core active, and the shoulders stabilized.

2. Partner A extends the legs back, tucking the toes under, while keeping the arms and legs straight, shoulder blades together and chest open, neutral alignment through the torso, and hips level.

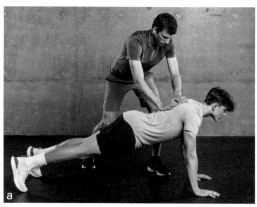

3. Partner B places both hands evenly on partner A's upper back.

4. Partner A performs a push-up, lowering the chest toward the floor then pressing the hands into the floor to return to the start position.

5. Partner B adds slight resistance with the hands against both the press up and on the lowering down of the push-up.

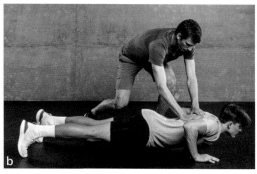

6. Repeat for reps and then switch roles.

Tips and Variations

- If too much pressure is used, partners will not be able to complete the sets; communicate with your partner to determine the correct level of resistance to apply.

- To make the movement easier, lower into a kneeling push-up.

SIDE PLANK HOLD

Adding rotational movements into any workout is an excellent way to train functionally. In everyday life, we move and twist on a regular basis; therefore, training how we live is an effective way to stay fit and decrease the risk of injuries.

Equipment

- Mats (2; optional)

Movement Cues

1. Partners begin in a side-by-side forearm plank position; the elbows are under the shoulders, the legs extended, and the toes tucked under. Keep the core active, hips level, and the torso in a neutral position.

2. To accommodate differences in partner heights, start with the elbows in line on the floor.

3. Partners need enough room to rotate into a side plank in both directions so adjustments in positioning may be necessary.

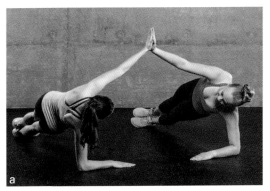

4. To begin, both partners rotate to their outside arms so they face each other.

5. In tandem, Partner A lifts the left arm and partner B lifts the right arm, extending the arms to touch their hands together.

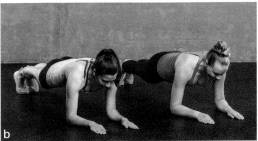

6. Add equal pressure to the hands and hold for 1-2 seconds.

7. Transition back into the forearm plank and immediately rotate to the inside arm, back-to-back, lengthening into a straight-leg plank. Extend the opposite arms to the ceiling, and touch the back of the hands together.

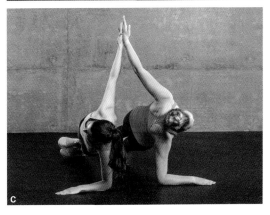

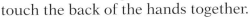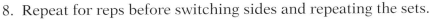

8. Repeat for reps before switching sides and repeating the sets.

Tips and Variations

- If a straight-leg plank is too challenging, opt for a kneeling plank or a modified plank with one knee bent and the opposite leg extended.

- To increase the challenge, hold the hands together at the top for two to four seconds before returning to the plank position.

- Once the skill is mastered, make the movements harder by increasing the speed of the rotating planks.

MODERATE

ROTATING SIDE PLANKS

The side plank is just one variation in a very large collection of plank options. When planking from the side, you can make the move easier or more challenging based on the position of the legs and arms, or the amount of contact with the floor.

Equipment

- Mats (2; optional)

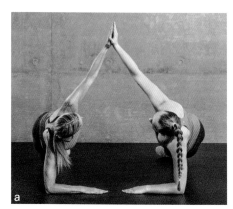

Movement Cues

1. Partners begin lying on one side, facing each other.

2. With the feet and the legs stacked or slightly staggered, lift the bottom hip off the floor to draw the side of the body up, and position the elbow directly under the shoulder and the forearm perpendicular to the torso.

3. Keep the core active and the torso in neutral alignment.

4. Both partners extend the top arm straight up and aligned with the chest, reaching to the ceiling.

5. Partners bring their extended hands together and press as hard as possible, without pushing each other over.

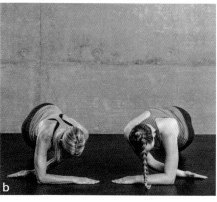

6. Hold for two to three seconds, then release and draw the extended arm down, rotating through the torso to sweep the arm under the body while reaching to the floor behind the body.

7. Reverse the rotation and reach up again to meet your partner's hand and hold this position.

8. Repeat for reps before resting and switching to the other side.

Tips and Variations

- To make the side plank easier, drop down to the knees or scissor the feet farther.

- To increase the challenge, perform the exercise as a straight-arm side plank and lift the top leg to be level with the hip.

RESISTED OBLIQUE CURL

Training the obliques is important for strengthening the midsection in flexion and rotation. The internal and external obliques work together to help us flex and bend. In this exercise, the obliques are challenged by the addition of partner resistance placed on the shoulder of the exerciser.

EASY

Equipment

- Mat (1; optional)

Movement Cues

1. Partner A begins by lying on the floor with partner B standing or kneeling.

2. Partner A gets into an abdominal curl position with the knees bent, the feet flat on the floor, the hands behind the head, and the core engaged.

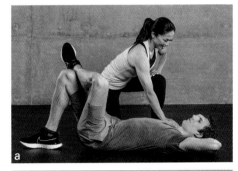

3. Partner A crosses the left foot over the right thigh, forming a figure-four shape.

4. Partner B kneels beside partner A with the inside (right) knee down and the left foot on the floor, and places an open right palm on partner A's right

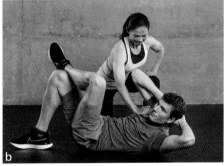

upper chest just parallel to bottom of the arm pit and up toward the shoulder.

5. Lifting the head, the neck, and the shoulders off the floor, partner A rotates the right shoulder toward the left knee, keeping the gaze forward and the chin slightly tucked in, while partner B adds resistance to partner A by pressing against the chest as partner A curls up.

6. There should be enough pressure for partner A to feel the obliques contracting, but not so much that partner A cannot lift up.

7. Partner A repeats for reps, switches to the other side, and then the partners switch roles.

Tips and Variations

- Allow the partner to practice a few reps before adding resistance if this is the first time performing the exercise together.

- The goal is to have just enough resistance that it can be felt, but not so much that the partner can't lift the head and shoulders off the floor.

- It is important to communicate in this exercise to find the correct level of resistance.

CHAPTER 7

Small-Equipment Exercises

In this chapter, partners will incorporate either a resistance band or a medicine ball into the training format. Adding equipment has many benefits. Equipment can intensify exercises and can even act as a buffer. Plus, equipment adds a fun twist to certain movements by making them interesting and challenging. Choose a variety of weights for the medicine balls, if available, or try different styles of weighted balls like a plyo ball or slam ball (see more details in chapter 3). An assortment of resistance bands with varying thicknesses is ideal as well, especially if partners are at different fitness levels. Always inspect the resistance bands and ensure they have no tears or rips before beginning your workout.

SQUAT TO SIDE PASS

Sometimes the simplest exercises are the best exercises. In this drill, the medicine ball is passed laterally from partner to partner. For an added balance challenge, partners stand on one leg. When possible, add some balance work to base moves to develop your body control. As we get older, falls become more common so staying strong and working on balance will help decrease the risk.

Equipment

- Medicine ball or plyo ball

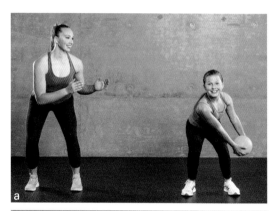

Movement Cues

1. Stand shoulder to shoulder, facing the same direction.

2. Move apart from each other in the same line, approximately six or more feet.

3. Holding onto the medicine ball at chest level, partner A drops down into a squat, rotating the medicine ball to the outside knee, then drives up through the legs to return to standing while passing the ball to partner B, who catches it.

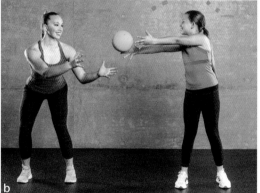

4. Partner B drops into a squat, rotating the medicine ball to the outside knee, and then drives up through the legs to return to standing while tossing the ball back to partner A.

5. After a few practice tosses, increase the challenge by balancing on the inside leg and continue the squatting, lifting, and tossing action.

6. Complete for reps and then switch sides with your partner to toss from the opposite direction.

Tips and Variations

- To make the movement easier, avoid squatting too low or stay closer to your partner.

- To increase the challenge, use a heavier medicine ball, stand farther apart, or increase the tempo of the passes.

WOODCHOPPER

The wood chop is an exercise training staple. Generally the movement travels across the body from a high to low position, but in this set, the motion is performed in the opposite direction, from low to high, as well. The diagonal pattern of this movement activates both the internal and external oblique muscles.

Equipment
- Medicine ball or plyo ball

Movement Cues
1. Stand back-to-back, with partner A holding the medicine ball.
2. Both partners drop into a squat, with the feet wider than shoulder-width apart, the core engaged, the knees bent, and the torso long.
3. Partner A holds the medicine ball with both hands below the right hip, then lifts up the ball diagonally across the body and passes it over the left shoulder to partner B.
4. Partner B receives it from near the top of the right shoulder and brings it down diagonally across to below the left hip, to pass it to partner A's right side below the hip.
5. The movement continues in a smooth rotation from low to high and high to low in both directions, and repeating for reps.

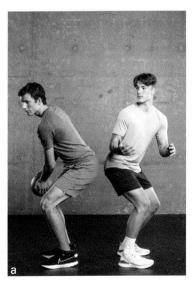 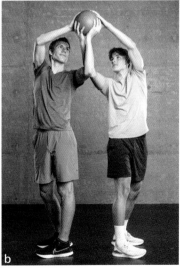

Tips and Variations
- To increase the challenge, use a heavier medicine ball, increase the passing speed, or get lower into the squat.
- Partners can also step slightly farther apart, requiring more of a reach to pass and receive the ball.

FORWARD AND BACKWARD LUNGE AND PASS

Lunges are a favorite lower body exercise because they work the glutes, quads, hamstrings, and calf muscles. Lunging forward and backward requires balance and coordination. If you find it difficult to balance, focus your gaze on a spot on the floor and keep the core very active. Control the movement through the start to the finish.

Equipment

- Medicine ball or plyo ball

Movement Cues

1. Stand facing each other approximately two to three feet apart with right shoulders in line and partner A holding a medicine ball.
2. In this movement sequencing, one partner lunges forward while the other partner lunges back.
3. To perform a lunge correctly, start in an upright position with the feet hip-width apart and the toes pointing forward.
4. Maintain a neutral spine position, the shoulders relaxed, and the chest open.
5. Step one leg behind, placing the back toes on the floor and bending the front knee to approximately 90 degrees.
6. Press the feet into the floor to push up into standing position, before stepping the same leg into a forward lunge.
7. In the forward lunge, keep the front knee behind the toe and bend the back knee to 90 degrees.
8. As partner A steps forward with the right foot, partner B steps backward with the left foot.
9. At the bottom of the lunge, partner A hands the medicine ball to partner B before they both push off and return to the start position.
10. Repeat the lunges and ball passes for reps before switching sides.

Tips and Variations

- To make the movement easier, perform a modified lunge or pass a lighter ball.
- To increase the challenge, move farther away from each other, pass a heavier medicine ball, increase the lunge speed, or increase the lunge depth.

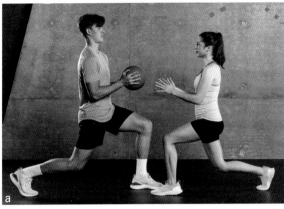

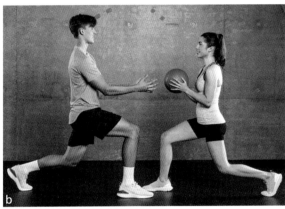

LATERAL LUNGE AND TOSS

Side or lateral lunges are a good alternative to the basic lunge and can be done with or without weight. Adding a reach and a medicine ball toss improves hip strength and mobility and rotational strength, and it will increase heart rate with the alternating side-to-side movement.

Equipment

- Medicine ball or plyo ball

Movement Cues

1. Stand facing each other approximately four feet apart.
2. To get warmed up, each partner takes a large step with the outside leg, dropping into a lunge position by pressing the hips back, keeping the core active, bending the outside knee, and keeping the inside leg straight.

MODERATE

3. It is important to keep the upper body upright and keep the knee behind the toe of the bent leg.

4. Repeat the lunge again, checking body position and getting used to the movement pattern.

5. Partner A picks up the medicine ball and both partners return to the start position, standing next to each other.

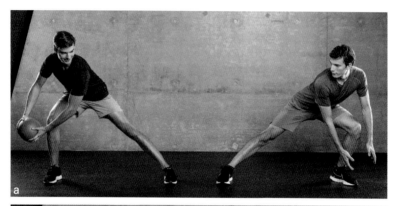

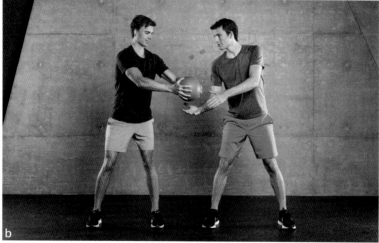

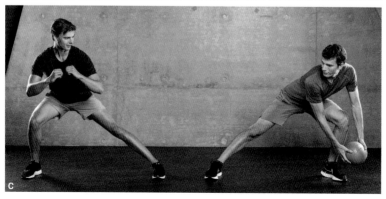

6. On the lunge to the right, partner A brings the medicine ball to the right knee or lunges low enough to touch the ball to the floor, then underhand passes the ball to partner B as partner A returns to the start position.

7. Partner B catches the ball and follows the same movement pattern, lunging laterally to the left, moving the ball to the left knee or touching it down on the floor, then passing it back to partner A.

8. Repeat the sets, continuing to mirror each other in the opposite direction, before partners switch sides.

Tips and Variations

- To make the movement easier, perform modified lunges, and slow down the movements.

- Another way to make the movement easier would be for one partner to lunge while catching and passing, while the other partner remains in the start position and only catches and passes.

- To increase the challenge, choose a heavier medicine ball, increase the tempo, or move farther apart from each other so you have to toss the ball farther.

BALL SLAM

Pent-up energy? This exercise is a perfect stress reliever. In this drill, it is preferable to choose either a plyo ball or slam ball. A plyo- or slam-style ball will squish into the surface where it lands and not move. If a medicine ball is used, be cautious. When thrown on the floor, a medicine ball tends to bounce and could potentially bounce up and cause injury.

Equipment

- Medicine ball or plyo ball

Movement Cues

1. Stand facing each other and far enough apart to catch the bounce of the medicine ball or to pick up a plyo ball.

2. Partner A holds the medicine ball in front of the waist and quickly lifts it high overhead, extending through the arms, then slams it straight down as hard as possible onto the floor, sinking into the hips to create more force.

3. Once the ball lands, partner B either catches the medicine ball on the bounce, or picks the ball off the floor if using a plyo ball.

4. Partner B then raises the ball overhead and throws it straight down onto the floor, where it is caught or picked up by partner A.

5. As an option, partner A can repeat the exercise for reps with partner B passing the ball each time to partner A, and then switching.

MODERATE

Tips and Variations

- Be careful when throwing a medicine ball; check how much bounce the ball has and make sure the floor surface is flat.
- To increase the challenge, use a heavier ball, lift it higher, or throw it down harder.
- Repeating the reps quickly will also make the exercise more challenging.
- If available, try a heavy plyo ball, so there is no bounce and each partner works more by picking up a heavy ball and passing it.

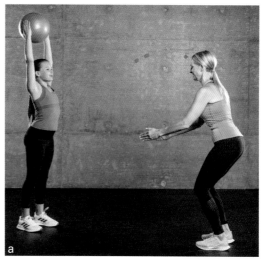

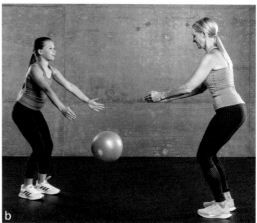

MODERATE

UNEVEN PUSH-UP AND ROLL

Adding a medicine ball to a push-up sequence adds variety and challenge. Choose a basic or more difficult push-up position. Partners can vary their choice of push-up to match their ability (see more in the Tips and Variations section). This exercise can be performed with one medicine ball or two. Make sure that the ball rolls easily.

Equipment

- Medicine ball(s); one or two (not a plyo ball)
- Mats (2, optional; for kneeling push-ups)

Movement Cues

1. Partners begin in a straight-arm plank position, facing each other, then each puts a medicine ball under the right hand.
2. Keeping the shoulders level, the body long, and the core engaged, both partners lower down into a push-up with the right hand resting on the medicine ball.

3. Return to the start position and roll the medicine ball directly across to your partner's left hand.

4. With the medicine ball under the left hand, both partners perform another push-up.

5. Continue for reps.

6. If there is only one medicine ball, partner A starts with the medicine ball under the right hand as both partners perform a push-up in tandem. At the top of the push-up, partner A rolls the ball straight across to partner B's left hand. Both partners perform the next push-up, and partner B rolls the ball on a diagonal to partner A's 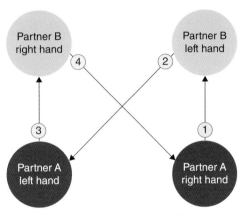 left hand. After the next push-up, partner A rolls the ball straight across to partner B's right hand, performs a push-up, and partner B rolls the ball on a diagonal to partner A's right hand. Repeat the sequence for the remaining repetitions.

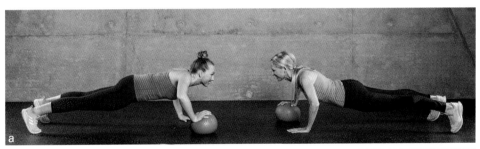

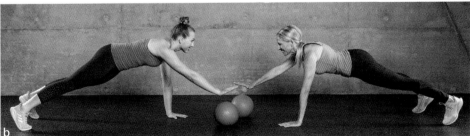

Tips and Variations

- To make the movements easier, perform the exercise in a kneeling push-up position.
- To increase the challenge, speed up the tempo of the sets.
- The medicine ball can be any weight but if using two balls, they should be the same diameter.

CURL-UP AND PASS

Combining the abdominal curl with a medicine ball pass makes a mundane abdominal exercise more interesting and effective. Always start with an easy medicine ball pass versus throwing the ball.

Equipment

- Medicine ball or plyo ball
- Mats (2; optional)

Movement Cues

1. Sit facing each other, knees bent, with the heels resting on the floor, and toes pointing up. The ankles can be overlapping or the feet can be farther apart.
2. To warm up, both partners roll down and back up, focusing on lowering and curling through the spine one vertebra at a time. After practicing a few rolls, add the medicine ball to the exercise.
3. Partner A holds the ball close to the body at chest height, and rolls all the way down to the floor. At the same time, partner B rolls down to the floor without a ball.
4. As both partners curl back up, partner A chest passes the ball to partner B, who catches it and rolls down holding the ball; partner A rolls down without a ball.
5. Both partners repeat the set and at the top of the curl, partner B passes the ball back to partner A.

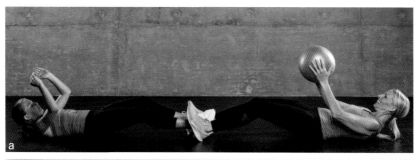

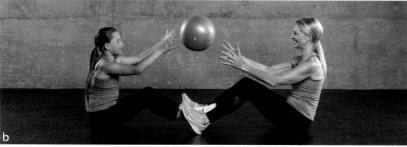

Tips and Variations

- To increase the challenge, choose a heavier medicine ball or move farther apart.
- Another progression is to hold the medicine ball farther away from the body on the roll down (i.e., hold the ball with straight arms in front or over the head).
- To engage more of the abdominals and core, attempt to toss the ball from above the head (overhead pass) versus a chest pass.

SIT AND PASS

The sit and pass exercise is a great way to get your core involved while strengthening your upper body. As you progress in the exercise, incorporate different weighted medicine balls or move farther away from your partner to make the exercise more or less challenging. Additionally, increase the passing tempo between you and your partner, speeding up the throwing and catching sequence.

Equipment

- Medicine ball or plyo ball
- Mats (2; optional)

Movement Cues

1. Sit facing each other with the feet on the floor and the toes touching; the knees are bent and the trunk is at an approximate angle of 45 degrees.
2. Keep the core engaged by bracing the abdominal muscles, pulling in and down.
3. To position correctly, both partners extend their arms forward; with their arms outstretched, the fingers should just barely touch.
4. Partner A passes the medicine ball into partner B's outstretched hands, trying to keep the trunk still.
5. Partner B immediately passes the ball back to partner A.
6. Once each partner is used to the weight of the medicine ball and the passing motion, move farther away from each other so that you have to throw the ball into your partner's hands.
7. Repeat the exercise for reps.

MODERATE

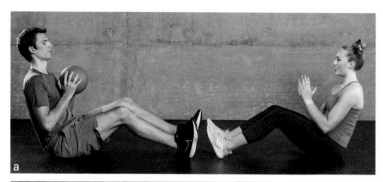

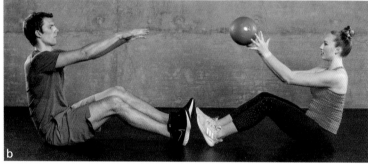

Tips and Variations

- If the extended seated position is uncomfortable for either partner, modify the body position by sitting up taller or by sitting on a rolled-up towel that is placed under the glutes.
- Always begin by passing the ball before progressing to throwing.
- Make sure the passes are very accurate to avoid catching a ball anywhere other than directly in front of you.

SEATED PASS WITH ROTATION

Working the abdominals with a partner is a fun and effective way to rev up the midsection. The variation and challenge in this exercise is attributed to how heavy the medicine ball is and the tempo with which the ball is passed.

Equipment

- Medicine ball or plyo ball
- Mats (2; optional)

Movement Cues

1. Sit side by side on the floor, facing the same direction with knees bent.

MODERATE

2. To position correctly, partners slightly turn their torsos toward each other and extend their arms; with the arms outstretched, the fingers should just barely touch.

3. The feet are on the floor, and the trunk is in a neutral position, leaning back at a comfortable, but challenging, angle.

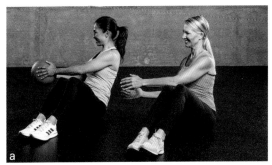

4. The core is engaged and the abdominal muscles are braced, pulling in and down.

5. Partner A picks up the medicine ball and taps it on the floor on the outside hip.

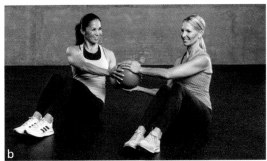

6. Partner A passes the ball to partner B, who then rotates the ball to the outside hip and taps the floor before passing it back.

7. Repeat the back-and-forth motion for reps before switching sides.

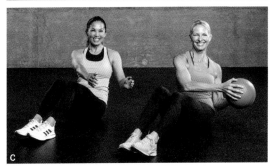

Tips and Variations

- To make the movement easier, partners can sit closer together and gently pass the ball.
- Other less intense modifications include passing a lighter ball, not rotating as far to the side, and sitting up taller versus leaning back.
- To increase the challenge, move farther away from each other and throw the medicine ball versus passing it.

HARD

SKIER

This exercise sequence combines two movements: press backs and side-to-side hops. One partner is active in the exercise sequence and the other acts as an anchor. However, because of the high challenge level of the drill, having a back-and-forth work–recovery pattern is ideal.

Equipment

* Resistance band (1)

Movement Cues

1. Stand face-to-face.
2. Partner A takes hold of both handles of the band and partner B holds the band in the center with both hands, palms down.
3. Partner B draws the elbows back, forearms hugging the sides, and holds the band secure at approximately waist height.
4. Partner A steps away from the anchor point until there is tension on the band, holding the handles with the arms extended down at the sides and the palms facing back.
5. Partner A bends the knees slightly, hinges at the hips, keeping the spine neutral and hands at the sides and slightly back.

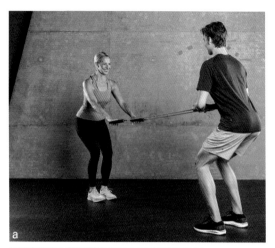

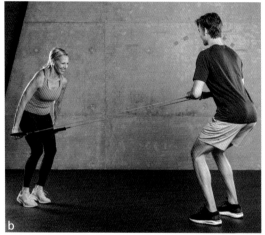

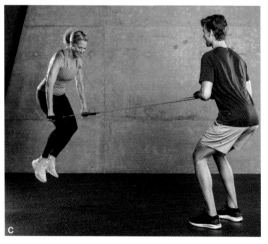

6. Partner A presses the arms behind and up in a posterior position.

7. As the arms lift behind, partner A hinges at the hips to drop the chest toward the floor, continuing to press the arms up.

8. Partner A returns to a semi-upright position, with the arms at the sides.

9. To progress, partner A increases the tempo of the movement of the upper body and hops from side to side. The feet stay together with each press back of the arms for a challenging cardio burst.

10. Repeat for time before switching roles.

Tips and Variations

- To make the exercise easier, choose to do the press backs only, or use a thinner resistance band.

- To increase the challenge, accelerate the tempo of the movement, use a thicker resistance band, or make the side-to-side jumps bigger.

FOOTBALL RUN

The football run may be used in the warm-up at a slower and longer tempo, or as a high-intensity interval training exercise within a circuit or cardio program. This exercise is ideal for improving agility and coordination. Initially, one partner may start while the other partner is the timer. After the first set, the roles switch. This allows each partner to have a rest between work sets.

Equipment

- Resistance bands (2)

Movement Cues

1. Place the resistance bands on the floor, forming an X.

2. Partners face each other standing within each side of the X.

3. Start by stepping each foot from the inside to the outside of the band, right (R) foot, then left (L) foot.

4. Immediately step back in, R foot, then L foot to continue the RLRLRL pattern.

5. Practice the out-out-in-in movement at a slow pace.

6. Once the footwork is mastered, without stepping on the band, increase the pace.

7. Step the feet out and in as fast as possible, moving the arms in a running-like pattern.

8. Repeat for reps with the opposite leg leading.

MODERATE

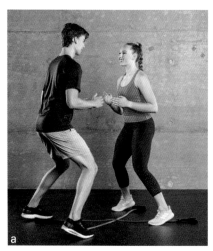 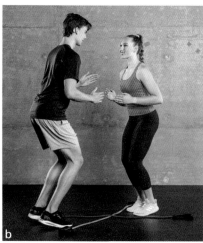

Tips and Variations

- The tempo chosen should be based on the fitness level of each partner; the faster you move, the more challenging it is.
- Alternate each set with your partner or move in tandem.
- In round one, lead with your right foot; in round two, lead with your left foot.
- As skill improves, make sure the arms are working in combination with the legs.

SIDE SHUFFLE

Shuffling from side to side is a great way to build speed and agility, and will especially benefit anyone who plays sports. Because we spend the majority of our time moving forward and backward, lateral movement training ensures that we train in various planes of movement.

Equipment

- Resistance band (1)

Movement Cues

1. Stand shoulder to shoulder facing the same direction.
2. Partner A begins by wrapping the band around the waist and looping the right handle through the left handle, pulling it snug across the hips.
3. The length of the remaining band is pulled to the right side of the body and held by partner B.

MODERATE

4. Once in position, partner B squares up and faces the side of partner A.

5. Partner B maintains an athletic ready position, with the knees slightly bent and the core active, holding the handles tightly.

6. Partner A lowers the body slightly and begins to shuffle to the left, pulling against the tension of the band.

7. Traveling as far as possible, partner A reaches down and touches the floor with the left hand before shuffling back to the start position.

8. Complete for reps or time, shuffling quickly and touching the floor with the hand.

9. Repeat the movements in the opposite direction by moving the band and switching to the opposite side.

10. Switch partner roles.

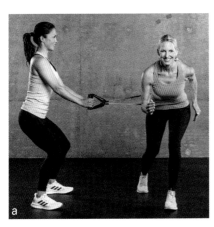 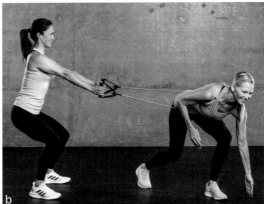

Tips and Variations

- Position the band so that it doesn't slip during the shuffle: Ensure the band is low enough on the hips; it may be necessary for the person shuffling to hold the band in one place. If so, hold with the hand that is not touching the floor.

- To increase the challenge, choose a thicker resistance band, travel farther from the anchor point, or shuffle faster.

PARACHUTE BAND RUN

Being able to increase your lower body strength through running and jumping is an effective way to get stronger and improve your cardio conditioning with a heart rate boost. Running with speed parachutes is popular with athletes. Instead of the drag of a parachute, try the resistance of the band to make you work harder and get stronger.

Equipment

- Resistance band (1)

Movement Cues

1. Partner A places the center portion of the resistance band around the hips.
2. Partner B stands behind partner A while holding a handle in each hand, and walks back until there is slight tension on the band.
3. Partner B maintains an athletic ready position or offset stance with the knees slightly bent, the core active, and the resistance band handles held tightly.
4. Partner A runs forward as far as possible until reaching maximum tension on the band, as partner B anchors the band.
5. At the highest tension point, partner A may choose to hold against the resistance while high-knee running in place before returning to the start position.
6. After repeating for reps or time, switch roles.

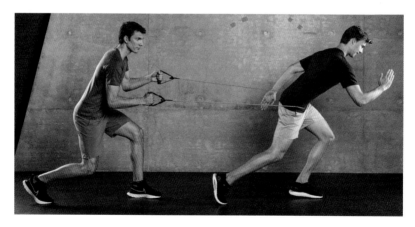

Tips and Variations

- Ensure that the band is low enough on the hips so it doesn't slip. It may be necessary to hold the band in one place; if so, alternate from a right- to left-hand hold after each resisted run.
- To increase the challenge, choose a thicker resistance band.

FRONT PRESS AND LEAP

The chest press and leap combined with the pull from the band is challenging and effective. Combination movements as shown in this exercise, are ideal for whole body integration. This exercise has a two-step exercise progression that requires coordination with your partner.

Equipment

- Resistance band (1)

Movement Cues

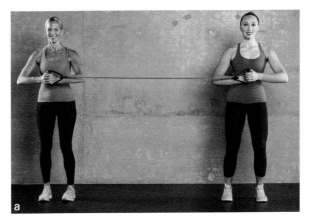

1. Stand shoulder to shoulder with your partner, facing the same direction, and each holding one end of the band with both hands and elbows bent.

2. Partners move apart from each other until there is tension on the band.

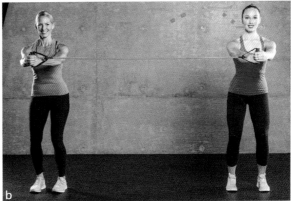

3. Holding the handles close to the body at chest height, hop forward and slightly to the side (away from each other) while pressing and extending the hands forward at the same time.

4. Pause for 1-2 seconds then return to the start by hopping back and bringing the hands back to the chest.

5. Work together by communicating with your partner when to jump and press.

6. Complete for reps before switching sides.

Tips and Variations

- To make the movement easier, replace the leap with a giant step.
- To increase the challenge, try leaping farther to the side, extending the arms farther, holding longer and leaping back to the start position.
- To increase the challenge even more, accelerate the tempo of the movement.

MODERATE

LONG JUMP

In this exercise, one partner performs the exercise while the other partner is the anchor and creates the resistance. The resistance band rests around partner A's hips as they jump forward as far as possible.

Equipment

- Resistance band (1)

Movement Cues

1. Partner A places the center portion of the resistance band around the waist.
2. Partner B stands behind partner A holding one end of the band in each hand and walks back until there is slight tension on the band.
3. Partner B maintains an athletic ready position with the knees slightly bent and the core active.
4. Partner A jumps as far forward as possible, performing a standing long jump.
5. To jump properly, partner A should focus on bending through the knees and using the arms to assist by creating momentum and exploding up and forward.
6. After sticking the landing, partner A walks back to the starting position and repeats.
7. Perform for reps and switch partner roles.

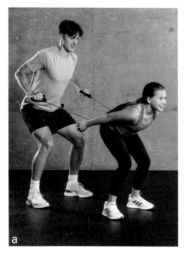 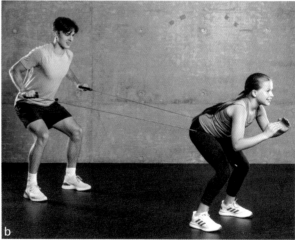

Tips and Variations

- Position the band so that it doesn't slip during the jump. Ensure the band is low enough on the hips; it may be necessary for the person jumping to hold the band in place. If so, alternate from a right- to left-hand hold after each jump.

- To make the movement easier, step forward as far as possible instead of jumping.
- To increase the challenge, attempt to jump farther, use a thicker or more challenging resistance band, or increase the tempo of each rep.

ROW AND HOP BACK

Exercises that focus on the back of the body help to balance all the time we spend on the front. Because the back tends to be fairly strong, don't shy away from choosing a thicker or more challenging resistance band. When performing rows, partners can work together simultaneously by looping multiple bands together.

Equipment
- Resistance band (1)

Movement Cues
1. Partner A holds both handles of the band and stands facing partner B.
2. Partner B becomes the anchor and takes hold of the center of the band with both hands, stepping away from partner A until there is moderate to heavy tension on the band, and maintains an athletic ready position with the knees slightly bent and the core active.
3. Partner A stands with the feet hip-width apart, hinging from the hips, the knees slightly bent, the core active, and the arms extended toward partner B.

MODERATE

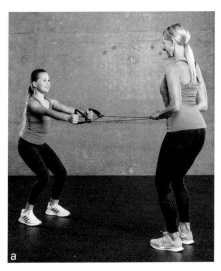
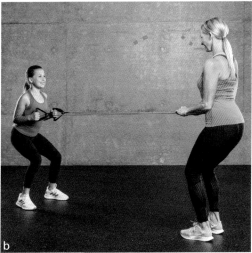

4. To perform the row, partner A pulls the handles back, contracting the mid- and upper back muscles to bring the arms close to the sides with elbows bent.

5. To add an additional layer of complexity, after completing the row and holding the arms close to the sides, back muscles contracted, partner A hops backward against the resistance and then hops forward before extending the arms and performing the next row.

6. Repeat for reps before switching roles.

Tips and Variations

• As an option, partners can perform the standing rows at the same time; using two bands, each person loops the bands in the center. Move away from your partner until there is tension on the band, and repeat steps 4-6.

• For variety, change the position of the arms from a low row (elbows low and close to the sides), to a moderate row (elbows slightly out from the sides of the body), or to a high row position (elbows to the sides at chest height).

LUNGE AND ROTATION

Stepping into the lunge while holding the arms in front at chest level and rotating is a multiplanar, full body movement. Adding a resistance band while moving at the same time as your partner further increases the balance challenge, the coordination, and the concentration needed to do the movement well.

Equipment

• Resistance band (1)

Movement Cues

1. Stand side by side facing the same direction, each holding one end of the resistance band in both hands.

2. Step away from each other to the side until there is light tension on the band.

3. Simultaneously, each partner lunges forward with their outside leg, keeping both knees bent at approximately 90 degrees, the core active, and the front knee in line with or behind the front toe. The front thigh should be parallel to the floor at the lowest point of the lunge.

4. Both partners lower into the lunge, extending the arms while holding the resistance band. Rotate the arms away from each other while keeping tension on the band.

5. Maintain proper alignment in the lower body while rotating through the upper body; there should be no twisting in the lower body.

6. Keep the core active during the rotation.

7. Return back to center and push with the front foot to return to the start position.

8. Repeat for reps and switch sides to repeat the exercise in the opposite direction.

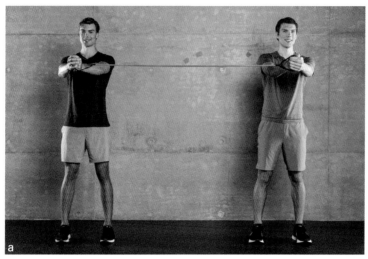

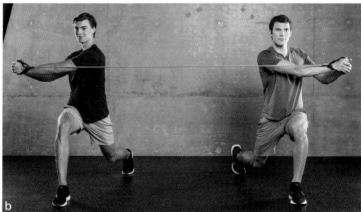

Tips and Variations

- To make the movements easier, break the exercise into separate parts: lunge, extend the arms, rotate, draw the arms back, and then return to the start position.

- To further modify, one partner performs the movement and the other partner acts as an anchor, then switch.

- To increase the challenge, ask your partner to step farther away to create greater resistance on the band, increase the tempo, or use a thicker or more challenging band.

CHEST PRESS

The chest press is a great exercise to work the pectoralis muscles and is a good alternative to the push-up. If only one band is available, one partner can serve as the anchor to the other (see notes in the Movement Cues section).

Equipment

- Resistance bands (2)

Movement Cues

1. Using two resistance bands, loop one band over the other creating a center anchor.
2. Stand facing away from each other while holding the handles of the resistance band, moving apart until there is tension on the bands.
3. In a staggered stance, each partner performs a chest press at the same time: Lift the arms up with the elbows bent at 90 degrees, keep the forearms parallel to the floor, and fully extend the arms to push the band forward in front of you.
4. Return to the start position by flexing the elbows and pulling the shoulder blades together.
5. Repeat the exercise for reps.
6. If only one band is available, the same exercise can be performed one partner at a time: Partner A stands holding both handles of the band in front of partner B, who becomes the anchor and takes hold of the center of the band with both hands, and then steps away from partner A until there is light tension in the band. Partner A

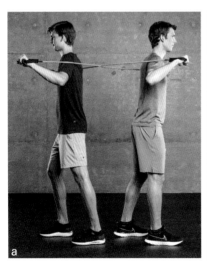
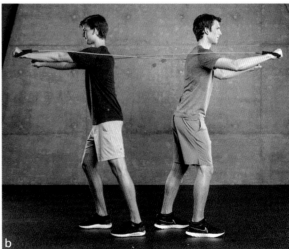

performs the chest press for the desired number of repetitions, then the partners switch.

Tips and Variations

- To increase the challenge for any of the chest press options, add in a lunge. Partners lunge away from each other, simultaneously pushing the band forward and stepping forward. Alternate left and right lunges.
- To further increase the challenge, step farther away to create greater resistance on the band, increase the tempo, or use a thicker or more challenging band.

BICEPS CURL AND SIDE LUNGE

MODERATE

Every day we lift objects or perform movements that use the biceps muscle. You can create different variations of the biceps curl exercise by tweaking the position or the type of resistance, allowing you to target the muscle group in different ways. In this biceps curl exercise, the resistance bands are hooked together.

Equipment

- Resistance bands (2)

Movement Cues

1. Using two resistance bands, loop one band over the other creating a center anchor.
2. Stand facing each other, holding the handles of the resistance bands, with the arms at the sides and the palms facing up.
3. Lift up both arms until they are parallel to the floor, and then flex and make an L-shape angle at the elbow. The partners move apart until there is tension on the bands.
4. In the start position, each partner performs a high biceps curl at the same time.
5. Return to the start position by extending the elbows and straightening the arms.
6. Once both partners are comfortable with the curl, add in a side lunge, moving in opposite directions from each other.
7. Alternate from one side to the other, all while performing the high biceps curls.
8. Repeat the exercise for reps.
9. If only one band is available, the same exercise can be performed one partner at a time: Partner A stands holding both handles of the band in front of partner B, while partner B becomes the anchor

and takes hold of the center of the band with both hands. Partner B then steps away from partner A until there is light tension in the band. Partner A performs the biceps curl and side lunge for the desired number of repetitions, then the partners switch.

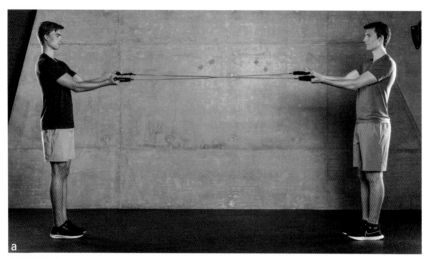

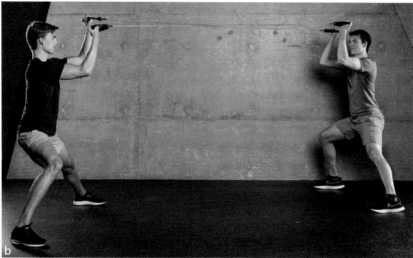

Tips and Variations

- To make the movements easier, use a thinner or less resistant band or eliminate the side lunge portion of the exercise.
- To increase the challenge, use a thicker or more challenging resistance band or step farther away from each other to create more tension.

HIGH ROW WITH WIDE SQUAT

A basic high row exercise works the muscles of the middle and upper back. With poor posture being a concern for many individuals due to inactivity or bad habits, such as slouching in front of our computers and smartphones, back exercises should be prioritized in most exercise sequences. This exercise is made exceptional by combining upper back and leg movements, creating a full body exercise.

Equipment

- Resistance bands (2)

Movement Cues

1. Using two resistance bands, loop one band over the other creating a center anchor.
2. Stand facing each other, with the palms down, while holding each handle of the resistance band.

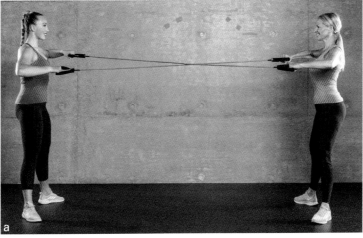

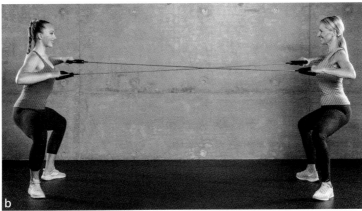

3. Lift and extend both arms until they are parallel to the floor, drawing the elbows slightly back. Partners move back from each other until there is light tension on the bands.

4. To begin, each partner performs a high row at the same time: Keep the chest lifted, draw the elbows back until the hands are right in front of the shoulders, and pull the shoulder blades together.

5. Return to the start position by straightening the arms.

6. Once both partners are comfortable with the high row, add in the wide squat: The feet are wide apart, the toes are slightly turned out, and the knees are in line with the feet as each partner lowers and lifts.

7. Repeat the row and the wide squat in sequence: lowering and pulling, and lifting and returning to the start at the same time.

8. If only one band is available, the same exercise can be performed one partner at a time: Partner A stands holding both handles of the band in front of partner B, who becomes the anchor and takes hold of the center of the band with both hands. Partner B then steps away from partner A until there is light tension in the band. Partner A performs the row and wide squat for reps, and then the partners switch.

Tips and Variations

- To make the movements easier, use a thinner band or eliminate the wide squat portion of the exercise.

- To increase the challenge, use a thicker resistance band, step farther away from each other to create more tension, or add an alternating and coordinated right and left side leg raise.

TRUNK ROTATION

Performing a rotation with a resistance band is a safe way to add challenge to a simple but effective exercise. Be sure to start slowly and proceed with control throughout the movement before increasing the tempo. Faster movements are fun and challenging, but rotation with speed should be done cautiously.

Equipment

- Resistance band (1)

Movement Cues

1. Face each other, with partner A holding both resistance band handles together, with the arms extended straight out and just under chest height.

2. Partner B holds the center of the band with both hands and acts as the anchor.

EASY

3. Step back from each other to create tension on the band; maintain an athletic ready position with a neutral spine, an active midsection, and a slight bend in the knees.

4. Partner A begins by rotating the extended arms to the right, back to center, then to the left, and back and forth.

5. Continue the rotations from side to side while keeping tension on the band, starting slowly and then going quickly from side to side without pausing in the center.

6. Repeat for time before switching roles.

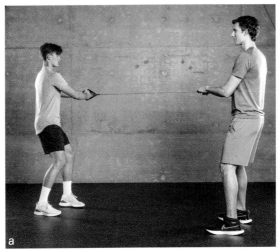

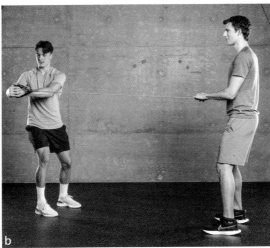

Tips and Variations

- Always move with control even when increasing and varying the tempo.
- To increase the challenge, choose a thicker resistance band or rotate the arms farther back, lifting the heels to pivot through the foot, lower body, and torso.

EASY

BOXING JABS

Boxing movements in a workout are excellent for improving upper body strength and speed. Using additional resistance provides a mechanism for not overextending through the elbow joint, and the amount of resistance can be adjusted by the distance from partner to anchor.

Equipment

- Resistance band (1)

Movement Cues

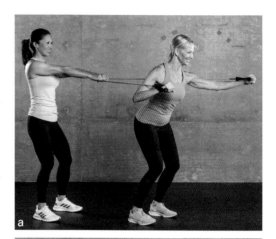

1. Partner A stands in front of and facing away from partner B, holding both handles of the band, with the rest of the band hanging loosely behind the back.

2. Partner B becomes the anchor and takes hold of the center of the band with both hands.

3. Partner B then steps back away from partner A until there is moderate tension on the band, maintaining an athletic ready position with the knees slightly bent and the core active, holding the center of the band securely.

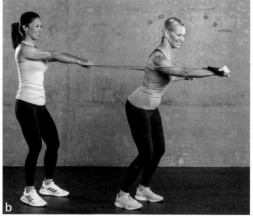

4. Partner A stands with the feet hip-width apart, squared up or in an offset stance, with the knees slightly bent and the core active.

5. Partner A raises the arms, elbows bent, almost parallel to the floor and at approximately chest level, making sure the band rests over the top of, and not under, the arms.

6. Partner A performs a punch with one arm then the other, alternating punches in front of the body, for a set time.

7. To complete the set, jab as fast as possible for the last 10 seconds.

8. Repeat for time before switching roles.

Tips and Variations

- When possible, try to adopt a boxer stance keeping the hands close to the chin and the elbows protecting the ribs.

- To increase the challenge, ask your partner to step farther back to create greater resistance on the band, or punch faster.

TRICEPS KICKBACK

To balance the front of the body, it is important to train the biceps counterpart, the triceps. Unlike the biceps muscles (biceps brachii or "bi's") located on the front of the upper arm, the triceps muscles (triceps brachii or "tri") make up the muscles on the back of the arm. Improving triceps strength provides stability to the shoulder and arms, and helps with movements like pushing and carrying things overhead and in sports like swimming.

Equipment

- Resistance bands (2)

Movement Cues

1. Using two resistance bands, loop one band over the other creating a center anchor.
2. Stand facing each other, with the palms down, while holding each handle of the resistance band.

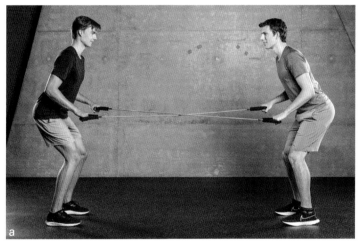

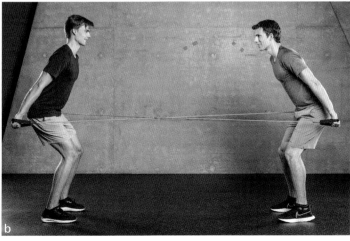

3. Partners step away from each other until there is slight tension on the bands and hinge forward slightly at the hips.

4. The arms are held close to the sides, the elbows bent at 90 degrees, and the palms facing the floor.

5. Both partners simultaneously extend the arms, bringing the hands slightly behind the hips.

6. Focus on contracting the triceps through the extension.

7. Return to the start position and repeat for reps.

Tips and Variations

- If only one band is available, the same exercise can be done either by working one arm at a time or by training one partner at a time. Option 1: Stand facing each other holding the handle of one resistance band. Repeat steps 3-7 for reps, before switching hands. Option 2: Partner A stands facing partner B who anchors the band by holding it in the center. Partner A holds onto one handle in each hand, hinges forward slightly, and presses the band back. Perform all repetitions, then switch partner roles.

- To increase the challenge, ask your partner to step farther back to create greater resistance on the band or increase the tempo.

TAP-DOWN ABS

Exercise enthusiasts appreciate new and unique ways to work the abdominals. The addition of the resistance band to the toe tap-down provides the needed intensity to fire up the abs and keep good movement control throughout the entire exercise.

Equipment

- Resistance band (1)
- Mat (1; optional)

Movement Cues

1. Partner A sits on the floor and loops the resistance band around the feet. Refer to the anchoring technique in table 3.1 found on page 26.

2. Partner A lies back and pulls the knees to the chest lifting the lower legs and feet.

3. Partner B stands in an athletic ready position at partner A's head and grasps the handles of the band.

4. Once positioned, partner A contracts the abdominals and lowers the feet slowly to the floor, tapping the toes on the floor.

5. Return to the start position and repeat for reps before switching roles.

MODERATE

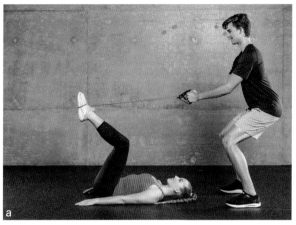

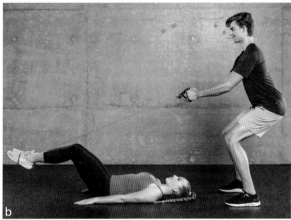

Tips and Variations

- It is important that the band be looped securely around the feet. Slightly point the toes down for added security.
- To make the movement easier, loop the band around one foot rather than both feet.
- To increase the challenge, partner B steps farther back so there is more resistance.
- A thicker resistance band will also make the exercise more challenging.

ROCK AND CURL

The rock and curl exercise combines multiple movements that maximize exercise results in less time. An abdominal curl is paired with a biceps curl, with each partner performing different movements simultaneously.

Equipment

- Resistance band (1)
- Mats (2; optional)

Movement Cues

1. Sit facing each other, the knees slightly bent, the heels on the floor with the feet together, and a slight lean back.
2. To warm up, both partners roll down and back up, focusing on lowering and curling through the spine one vertebra at a time. After practicing a few rolls, add the resistance to the exercise.
3. Partner A holds the handles of the band in each hand and extends the arms at chest level. Partner B becomes an anchor by holding onto the center of the band with the palms down and arms extended.
4. Partner A lifts the elbows, palms up and begins to roll down to the floor and performs a high biceps curl, pausing and holding the hands close to the shoulders.
5. Partner B proceeds to roll down to the floor simultaneously, and then both partners curl back up. Partner A extends the arms back to the start position and partner B maintains the anchor position.
6. Repeat the sequence for reps before switching roles.

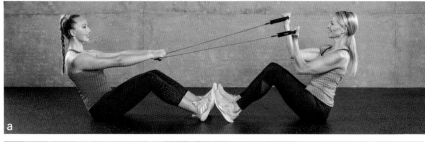

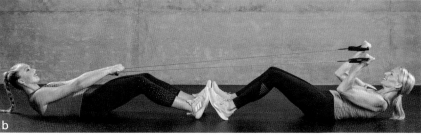

Tips and Variations

- To make the movements easier, the ankles can be overlapping so each partner is closer together creating less resistance on the band.
- To decrease the challenge, the partner anchoring the band remains in a semi-seated position versus curling down and up.
- To increase the challenge, use a thicker resistance band, slightly straighten the legs to move farther apart, or increase the tempo of the movements.

OBLIQUE BAND CURL

The obliques are important in flexing and rotating the spine. Unlike a straight curl-up that focuses on the rectus abdominus muscles, adding both rotation and resistance from the band fires up the internal and external oblique muscles. This exercise also allows each partner to train at the right intensity, meeting in the middle to create teamwork.

MODERATE

Equipment

- Resistance bands (2)
- Mats (2; optional)

Movement Cues

1. Sit facing each other on the floor, with the edge of partner A's right knee in line with partner B's left knee, and approximately one foot apart.
2. Each partner places a resistance band behind their back, underneath the arm pits and across their upper back, with the band length on the inside hand shorter than on the outside hand.
3. Partners set up in an abdominal curl position: lying on the back, the knees bent, the feet flat on the floor, and the band behind the back.
4. Partner A crosses the left foot over the right thigh, forming a figure-four shape.
5. Partner B crosses the left foot over the right thigh, forming a figure-four shape.
6. Partner A's right hand holds one end of the band at their right shoulder and their elbow is bent; the left arm is extended on the floor, holding and lengthening the other handle and creating a bit of tension on the band. Partner B's does the exact same position.
7. Lifting the head, the neck, and the shoulders off the floor, partner A rotates the right arm toward the left knee, keeping the gaze forward and chin slightly tucked in, as partner B does the same thing, both curling up to reach and meet hands in the middle.

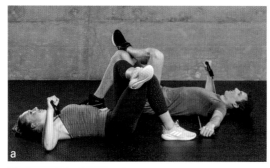

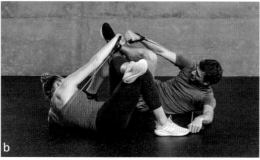

8. There should be enough pressure on the band to feel the obliques contracting, but not so much that you can't lift.

9. Repeat for reps and switch to the other side and then switch roles.

Tips and Variations

- Allow each partner to practice a few reps to ensure the right resistance on the band.

- The goal is to have just enough resistance that it can be felt, but not so much that either partner can't lift up the head and shoulders off the floor or extend the arm.

- It is important to communicate in this exercise to find the correct timing and connecting point.

- To make it harder or easier, adjust the band resistance. Shorten or lengthen the band or choose a thinner or thicker resistance band.

CHAPTER 8

Cardio and HIIT Exercises

High-intensity interval training (HIIT) is an efficient way to achieve more in a short period of time. As discussed in chapter 2, there are many benefits to interval training, especially using partner workouts. In this chapter, some of the exercises are done with or without equipment. Because intervals can be challenging, be sure to encourage your partner by cheering them on. Positive and motivational cues will be very beneficial.

With HIIT, always consider the work phase and the recovery phase. The work phase fluctuates based on the intensity, duration, and frequency of the high effort, with most intervals lasting around 30 seconds. The amount of recovery needed is based on the intensity of the interval. Choose passive recovery (very little movement) if the interval is extremely hard, or active recovery if the interval is less intense. High-intensity intervals are more fatigue causing and may require a longer recovery phase (e.g., 1:3, which means one minute of work and three minutes of recovery). The work-to-recovery ratio is generally dependent on the energy system focus during the work phase. Ultimately, the goal should be to complete the programmed work set at the highest intensity possible. Working extremely hard for only 15 seconds of a 30-second work set falls short of the interval goal. In this example, the overall work intensity should be adjusted in order to complete the 30-second goal.

To mix up the cardio sections, try one of the following HIIT formats with the exercises listed in this chapter:

- *Original Tabata:* 20 seconds of intense work, followed by 10 seconds recovery × eight sets. Total time: four minutes
- *Short modified Tabata:* 10 seconds of intense work, followed by 20 seconds recovery × eight sets. Total time: four minutes
- *Long modified Tabata:* 40 seconds of intense work, followed by 20 seconds of recovery for four to six sets. Total time: four to six minutes
- *Short intervals extreme:* 30 seconds of intense work, followed by 15 seconds of recovery × four sets. Total time: three minutes

- *Short intervals hard:* 30 seconds of hard work, followed by 30 seconds of recovery × four to six sets. Total time: four to six minutes
- *Long intervals:* 60 seconds to three minutes of intense work, followed by a recovery time equal to work time: 1:1, 1:1-1/2, or 1:2
- *Progressive intervals:* three sets of intervals increasing in intensity, followed by recovery. Building on the intensity of each set, there is no rest between sets. Duration is 60 seconds × three sets followed by a full recovery. The goal is to build an interval training base.
- *Pyramid intervals:* Increasing duration of intensity with the same recovery time between work sets. The length of time of the first work set determines the duration of the subsequent sets using a work-to-recovery ratio of 1:1, 2:1, and 3:1. The goal is to prepare for more challenging intensities while keeping the heart rate elevated throughout the work sets.

FOLLOW THE LEADER

The follow the leader drill can be used in a warm-up or as an interval-based cardio exercise. This exercise is ideal for improving agility, speed, and coordination. One partner is the leader and one partner copies, mirroring the movements. Start by facing each other and shuffling laterally side to side. Set the timer and after the set, repeat with partner B as the leader.

Movement Cues

1. Stand facing each other approximately two feet apart in an athletic ready position.
2. Decide who is going to lead, and who is going to follow, and pre-determine the duration of the set.
3. Partner A shuffles a few feet to the right, then to the left, as partner B attempts to mirror the movement.
4. Partner A can change the move, the tempo, and the direction of the movement as desired.
5. Continue for the duration of the set, then switch roles.

Tips and Variations

- Start with a slow tempo to get each partner used to shuffling laterally, side to side.
- The amount of space available will determine how far you can shuffle before changing direction.
- After the first set, try different movements such as jumping jacks, touching the floor, or moving backward.

EASY

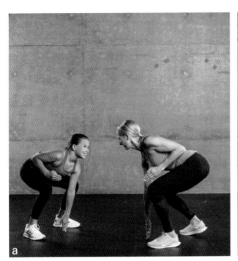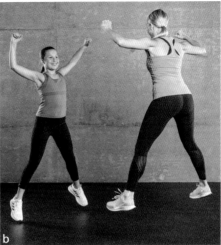

- The lead partner should not aim to completely lose the follower, but to choose simple movements and move at a pace that it is fun and cooperative.

HIGH-KNEES RUN

The high-knees run drill can be used in the warm-up or as a high-intensity interval training exercise. The partners are positioned facing each other and as they run in place, the goal is for the knees to tap the partner's outstretched hands. After one partner completes a set, rest before switching roles.

Movement Cues

1. Stand facing each other approximately two feet apart.
2. One partner creates the target and the other partner is running on the spot.
3. Partner A stands with the feet hip-width apart in a slight squat, arms extended, elbows bent, forearms parallel to the floor, and the hands out with palms down.
4. Partner B begins with a light march, working toward touching the knees to the palms of partner A's hands.
5. Once the target position is established, partner B can transition from a light jog to a high-knees run, aiming to touch the knees to partner A's palms each time.
6. Perform for time, then switch roles.

MODERATE

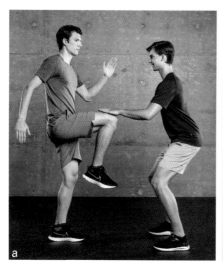
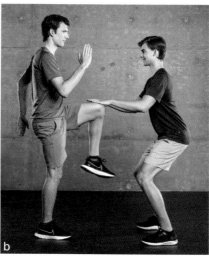

Tips and Variations

- The tempo chosen should be based on the fitness level of each partner; the harder you run, the more challenging the exercise is.
- Alternate each set with your partner; this allows one partner to rest while the other partner works.
- As skill improves, make sure the arms are pumping just as hard as the legs as you lift the knees.
- To make an easier target, lower the hands.
- To increase the challenge, lift the hands higher.
- For an interval challenge, repeat for three sets, transitioning from a longer interval to a shorter interval (i.e., 30 seconds, 20 seconds, then 10 seconds).

RESISTED RUN

This exercise is best executed when there is adequate space, such as a gym floor or an outdoor field, to maximize performance. The goal is to work cooperatively so that the drill is effective for both partners. The resisting partner should maintain appropriate pressure so the other partner is not unbalanced or falling. Working with a partner of similar size and strength is preferred if possible.

Movement Cues

1. Partners face each other, positioned in low, athletic ready positions.
2. Partner A repositions into an offset position with one foot forward and one foot back, hinging slightly at the hips and places both hands on the shoulders of partner B, adding light resistance.

HARD

3. Partner B begins to walk toward partner A while being resisted; once equal force and resistance are established, partner B tries to run toward the opposite side of the room as partner A resists the forward movement.

4. Continue for a set distance or time.

5. Switch positions and repeat with partner A running and partner B resisting.

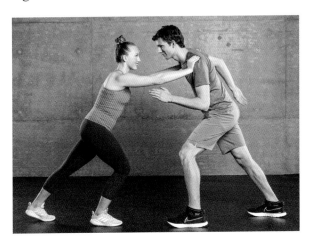

Tips and Variations

- The drill can be performed in a small space; however, both partners have to recognize how much pushing or resistance is needed in order to minimize the distance covered.

- Partners should provide enough resistance to make the exercise challenging, but not so much that the partner can't move or complete the exercise.

LEAPFROG

This old-school leaping drill is fun to use as a warm-up or as a workout drill. It requires space to execute it well, so a gymnasium or field is ideal.

Movement Cues

1. Partner A, facing away from and positioned about four feet in front of partner B, crouches with the hands and the feet on the floor, the knees tucked, and the head low.

2. Partner B jogs or runs to partner A, places the hands gently on partner A's back, and leaps over partner A's back.

3. Partner B runs forward about four feet and lowers into the crouching position so that partner A can leapfrog over.

4. Perform for time or distance.

MODERATE

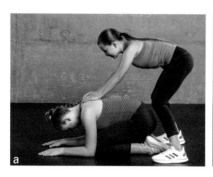 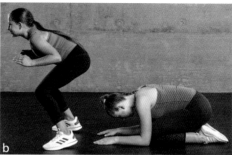

Tips and Variations

- It is important that partners trust each other.
- Partners should lightly press on each other's backs versus pushing down hard.
- To increase the challenge, partners can raise up slightly in the crouch position to make it more difficult to leapfrog over.
- Increasing the distance between each leap will also make the exercise more challenging, because you will run farther to leapfrog over your partner.

BURPEE JUMPS

This is a great combination drill that has both partners doing challenging exercises—burpees and back extensions—at the same time. It also requires coordination and timing.

Movement Cues

1. Partner A lies prone on the floor, the spine and the neck long and extended, elbows bent and head resting on the hands, and the legs extended straight back.
2. Partner B is positioned facing forward near one of partner A's hips, standing in an athletic ready position.
3. Partner B lowers the hips toward the floor into a partial squat and jumps over partner A's back, landing beside partner A's other hip.
4. Upon landing, partner B immediately performs a burpee by placing the hands on the floor, jumping the feet back into a plank, jumping the feet back in toward the hands, and standing up.
5. While partner B performs the burpee, partner A extends the spine, lifts the arms and legs off the floor, keeping the eyes looking down and the body long.
6. Partner A holds the back extension while partner B performs the burpee, returning the arms and legs to the floor as partner B jumps back over partner A.
7. Repeat the burpees and back extensions for a set amount of time before switching roles.

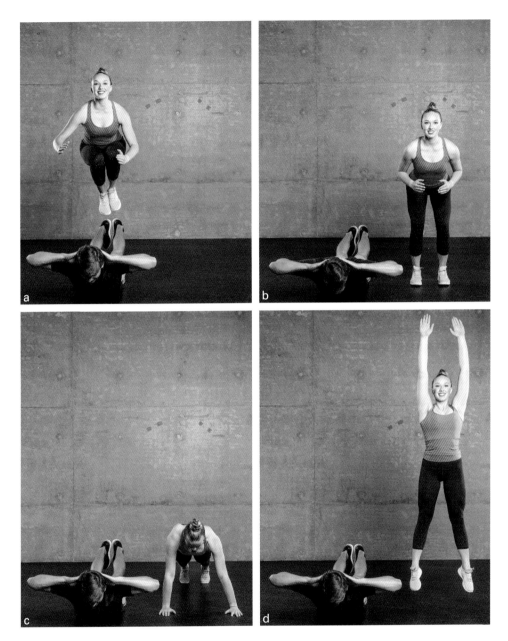

Tips and Variations

- The exercises can be performed side by side rather than with one partner jumping over the other.
- To make the burpee movement easier, step into the plank and back to the start position instead of jumping.
- To decrease the number of burpees in a set, partner B can leap over partner A three times and then perform one burpee, repeating the sequence with three leaps and one burpee.
- To increase the challenge, speed up the tempo of the jumps and burpees.

WIDE PLANK AND AGILITY FOOTWORK

In this core and agility exercise, both partners perform separate exercises but in combination. Correct footwork is an important component of this exercise and should be practiced first by both partners. This drill is ideal in the warm-up or as a cardio-based interval set.

Movement Cues

1. To learn the footwork, stand on the left foot with the right foot raised slightly off the floor. The movement pattern is to step down with the right foot and lift the left foot, step down with the left foot and lift the right foot, and step down with the right foot and lift the left foot and hold it up. Think, "right, left, right hold; left, right, left hold," or "run, run, hold" and repeat. Practice the agility move slowly, then speed up.

2. Once the footwork is perfected, add the plank: Partner A lowers into a high plank position with the hands under the shoulders, the legs extended back, and the feet positioned slightly wider than hip-width apart, keeping the body in neutral alignment from the shoulders to the toes. The shoulder blades are together, and the chest is open.

3. Partner B stands at partner A's left lower leg, facing the same direction.

4. Using the practiced footwork, partner B performs the agility work over partner A's lower legs. The "run run" happens to the inside of the legs and the "hold" happens outside partner B's legs. Travel from right to left and left to right.

5. After completing for time, partners switch roles and repeat the moves.

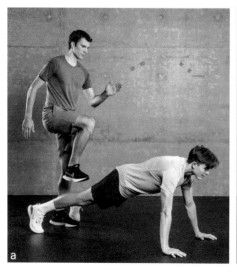 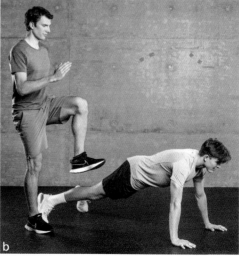

Tips and Variations
- The goal is to increase the speed of the agility work; however, start slowly and cautiously, especially when using the partner as a target.
- To make the footwork easier, walk the foot pattern, or perform the agility work beside each other versus over the top of each other.

PLANK LEAP

Getting more done in less time is the goal for most exercises. This combination drill is great for just that, because both partners perform challenging exercises—lateral jumps and a plank—at the same time. When jumping, there are options to do a two-foot side lateral jump, or a single repeating-leg leap.

Movement Cues
1. Partner A sets up in a forearm plank, elbows under the shoulders, legs extended back, core activated, feet positioned slightly wider than hip-width apart, and toes tucked under with the body in alignment from the shoulders to the toes.
2. Partner A remains in the plank for the entire set.
3. Partner B stands in an athletic ready position near one of partner A's hips, facing the same direction.
4. Partner B lowers into a partial squat and jumps explosively over partner A's back, landing on both feet near partner A's other hip.
5. Once landing, partner B immediately jumps back over to the other side, continuing for the set time, and then partners switch roles.

HARD

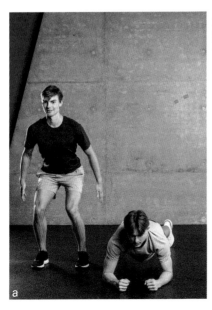
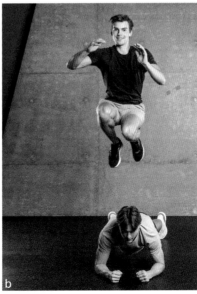

6. The other leaping option is a single-leg bound: Partner B lifts the foot closer to partner A's hip and jumps over partner A to land on the outside foot, keeping the other foot elevated. Partner B then jumps back to the start position, keeping one foot elevated.

Tips and Variations

- The exercises can be performed side by side, rather than one partner jumping over the other.
- To make the jumping easier, perform them over the planking partner's calves versus over the hips.
- To increase the challenge, either speed up the tempo of the jumps or hold a straight-arm plank rather than a forearm plank.

DONKEY KICK

For partners looking to add a creative spin to a traditional donkey kick exercise and maximize the challenge factor, this is just the exercise. Both partners need to be comfortable jumping over each other, and good communication is important.

Movement Cues

1. Partners stand beside each other facing the same direction.
2. Partner A gets into a plank: Start in a kneeling position with the hands under the shoulders and the core active. Walk the legs back until they are extended, tucking the toes under, and maintain neutral alignment through the torso with the hips level. The arms are straight with the hands under the shoulders, the shoulder blades are together, and the chest is open.
3. Partner B places both hands on the upper middle of partner A's back, with both feet together on the left side of partner A. Partner

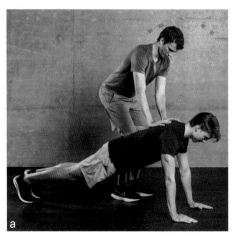
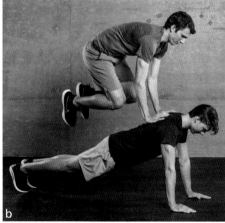

B bends the knees, lowers into a partial squat, and leaps up and over partner A's back.

4. Repeat the motion continuously, over and back, for reps before switching roles.

Tips and Variations

- To decrease the challenge, use a forearm plank as a less intense plank and a lower jump.
- To make the move even easier, switch out the plank for a tabletop position.

LONG JUMP AND HIGH JUMP

Both partners have an active role in this very physical exercise that combines jumping and more jumping. For the drill to be successful, there needs to be enough space for each partner to perform a long jump while facing each other.

Movement Cues

1. Partners stand facing each other about 10 feet apart.
2. Partners simultaneously lower the hips into a partial squat, drive the arms back and jump as far forward as they can, bringing the arms forward and performing a long jump.
3. Partners should land approximately two feet apart; adjust the start positions if needed.
4. Once the correct distance is determined, return to the start position and repeat the long jump.

HARD

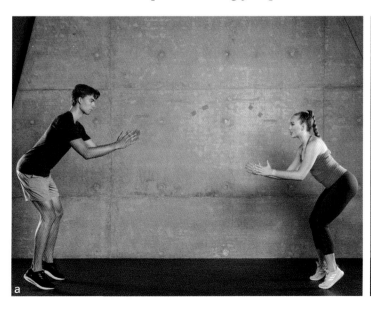
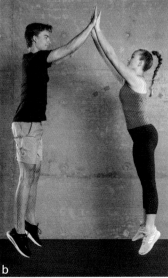

5. After landing the long jump, both partners jump straight up as high as possible and clap both hands together.

6. After landing the high jump, run backward as fast as possible to the start position.

7. Repeat the sets, focusing on jumping farther or higher each time.

Tips and Variations

- This exercise requires a learning curve to get the timing just right; practice slowly to begin and then increase the tempo as the skill level improves.

- To make the long jump easier, a partner could step as far forward as possible versus jumping.

- To increase the challenge, complete the high jump action three times before returning to the start position.

SQUAT JUMP TO HIGH 10

This exercise is an easy introductory partner move with minimal partner contact. It is a great exercise to use as a light warm-up, or it can be included in the interval part of the workout for a high-intensity burst.

Movement Cues

1. Partners stand facing each other, then step back about two to three feet apart.

2. The feet are approximately shoulder-width apart, the toes forward, and the knees in alignment with the feet. The spine is in a neutral position, and the head is in line with the spine, with the chin slightly tucked in. The arms are at the sides with the elbows bent.

   - Always maintain alignment by preventing the knees from shifting past the toes or collapsing inward or outward.

   - Keep the shoulders down and away from the ears.

3. Keep the core active, and bend the knees, the hips, and the ankles to lower into a squat.

4. Pressing through the feet, drive the glutes and the arms back, and explode with power to jump up as high as possible, extending the arms to the ceiling.

5. To coordinate the movement pattern with your partner, lower and jump at the same time, reaching up to give each other a high 10 with the hands at the top of the jump.

6. Repeat for reps or time.

HARD

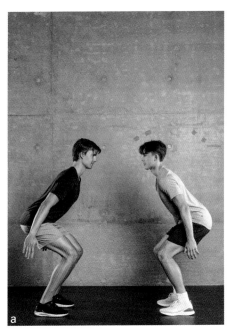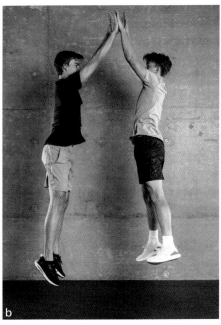

Tips and Variations

- Work in coordination with your partner to time the jumps.
- For a low impact option, skip the jump and adjust the movement as a squat to a standing position.
- To increase the challenge, squat lower, jump higher, or increase the tempo.
- As an option, start right shoulder to right shoulder and standing slightly apart; then lower into the squat and jump as high as possible high fiving the right hands together. After completing the reps, switch sides and repeat the jumps now high fiving with the left hands.

ROTATING SQUAT JUMP

This exercise utilizes speed, power, and coordination. It is a great one to use in the more challenging section of a warm-up, or it can be included in the interval section for a high-intensity burst.

Movement Cues

1. Stand shoulder to shoulder facing the opposite direction, then step about two to three feet apart. The feet are approximately shoulder-width apart, the toes forward, and the knees in alignment with the feet. The spine is in a neutral position, and the head is in line with the spine, with the chin slightly tucked in. The arms are at the sides with the elbows bent.

HARD

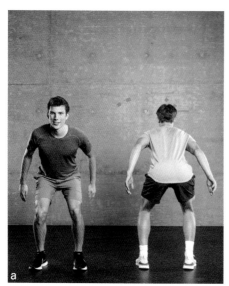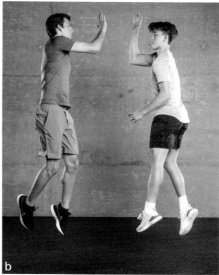

2. Keeping the core active, both partners bend the knees, the hips, and the ankles to lower into a squat, and each partner places the outside arm on the floor between the feet.

3. Pressing through the feet, drive the glutes and the arms back, and jump up powerfully, rotating a quarter turn to face your partner and give a high five with the outside hand.

4. After completing the reps, switch sides and repeat the jumps.

Tips and Variations

- For a low impact option, skip the jump and perform the movement as a squat to stand, and rotate the torso to give the high five to your partner.

- To increase the challenge, increase the jump rotation speed.

WALKOUT ANKLE TAPS

In this full body exercise, the goal is to move with both control and speed. It combines a hinge, walkout, and plank, and is a great exercise to use as a warm-up or full body move.

Movement Cues

1. Stand facing each other a little more than one full body-length apart.

2. Partner A hinges forward at the hips, keeping the legs straight, to lower the hands to the floor, moving the crown of the head toward the floor with the chin tucked in.

3. Once the hands reach the floor, partner A walks the hands forward into a plank position.

MODERATE

4. Partner A then taps partner B's left ankle with the right hand and partner B's right ankle with the left hand, before walking the hands back in toward the feet and standing up, keeping the legs straight the entire time.

5. Partner B now performs the exercise: hinging forward, walking out into a plank, and tapping partner A's ankles before returning to standing.

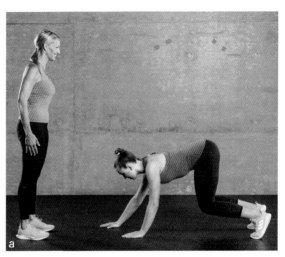

6. Adjustments to the distance may need to be made early in the sequence to ensure that each partner has to reach with an extended arm to tap the ankles.

7. Repeat for time, alternating partners each time.

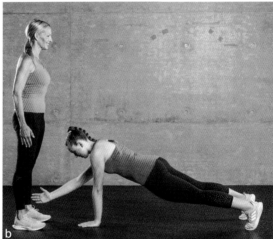

Tips and Variations

- As a progression option, hold the planks longer each time by increasing the number of ankle taps each set. For example, for first set, tap the R and L ankles and return to the start; second set, tap the ankles R, L, R, L and return to the start; third set, tap three sets of R, L, R, L, R, L ankle taps and so on.

- To increase the challenge, pick up the pace and try to complete as many as possible in a set amount of time.

- Another way to increase the challenge is to reach the hands up overhead in the standing position.

HARD

NARROW PUSH-UP AND HOP OVER

The push-up is a classic body-weight training exercise; it's a do-anywhere, do-anytime movement that strengthens the upper body and the core. Regardless of the variation or modification to the push-up, it is important to make sure that the spine is always in neutral alignment, the core is active, the head is in line with the spine creating a straight line, and the feet and hands are positioned correctly. Always lower only to the depth in which proper alignment can be maintained, and push the hands down into the floor when returning to the start position. Adding the two-foot hop over provides a cardioboost.

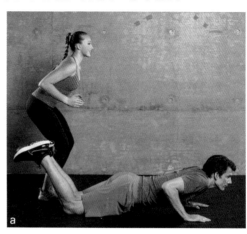

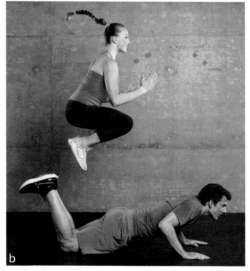

Equipment

- Mat (1; optional)

Movement Cues

1. Partner A begins in a straight-arm plank position, with the hands under the shoulders, legs walked back until they are extended, the feet positioned slightly wider than hip-width apart, the toes tucked under, the neutral spine position, and the core active. The shoulder blades are together, and the chest is open.

2. Partner B stands near partner A's lower right leg, facing the same direction as partner A.

3. Before lowering down from the plank position, partner A drops the knees down to the floor, lifts the feet, and shifts the body weight slightly forward.

4. Partner A tucks the arms in at the sides of the ribs and slowly lowers into a push-up, keeping the arms in close.

5. In the narrow position, keep the head in line with the spine, and then actively push into the floor to lift the upper body up.

6. Repeat the movement, focusing on good control.

7. As partner A lowers into the push-up, partner B lowers into a partial squat and explodes to jump up and laterally over partner A's legs.

8. Once on the other side, partner B touches the floor with the outside hand as partner A pushes back up to the top of the plank position.

9. As partner A lowers into another push-up, partner B leaps back over partner A's legs and touches the floor on the opposite side.

10. Repeat for jumps and push-up reps before switching partner positions.

Tips and Variations

- If partners prefer not to jump over each other, perform both exercises side by side.
- If the narrow position for the push-up is too challenging, opt for a wider hand position.
- To make the push-up more challenging, assume a fullbody position on the toes rather than on the knees.

CURL-UP AND JUMPING JACK

This exercise can be done with any partner combination. The strong position of the feet and hips on the floor provides a solid base. As an option, partners may choose to perform these exercises side by side versus on each other.

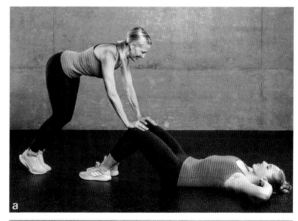

Equipment

- Mat (1; optional)

Movement Cues

1. Partner A lies faceup on the floor in an abdominal curl prep position: The knees are bent, the feet are placed flat on the floor approximately shoulder-width apart, and the head is resting in the hands.

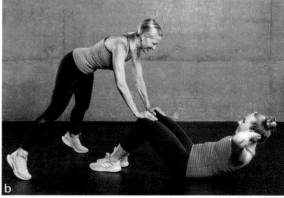

HARD

2. Partner B faces partner A and places the hands on partner A's knees and walks the feet slightly back.

3. Once in position with the hands lightly on partner A's knees, partner B hinges forward, keeping the back parallel to the floor and performs a jumping jack, jumping the feet out and in continuously.

4. Partner A maintains good alignment through the legs, and lifts the head and the shoulders off the floor,

5. The curls and the jacks continue in tandem for reps before partners switch roles.

Tips and Variations

- It is important that partners don't allow their legs to bow out to the sides in the curl-up position; the foundation needs to be strong.

- As an alternative to the jumping jack, perform a march, low run, mountain climber, or side-to-side hops.

- The exercise can also be done simultaneously, beside each other; replace the low jacks with standing jacks or a high-knees run.

- To increase the challenge, add an oblique curl; reaching the right elbow to the left knee, lowering down and lifting again to reach the left elbow to the right knee.

CHAPTER 9

Partner Solo Exercises

Working out with a partner can be done in a variety of formats. As fun as it is to be doing the same exercise as your partner, or using your partner as an exercise tool, it is not a realistic format for everyone. Partner workouts can still be creative and effective, even if you are not doing the exact same movements as your partner. In partner solo exercises, people with different skill sets or abilities can both be engaged and working out at the same time performing different exercises. For example, one partner could be doing burpees while the other partner does jumping jacks. Once the reps are completed, the partners switch exercises. Here are some exercises that pair well together.

JUMPING JACK

The jumping jack is a classic exercise that many of us may not have experienced since physical education classes from days past. Start with the feet together and the hands at the sides. Next, hop both feet out while lifting the hands overhead, hop the feet back in, and return the arms to the sides. Repeat the sequence. For a low-impact option, tap the toes right and left versus jumping. For an intermediate option, perform a plank-style jack with the hands on the floor and the feet hopping in and out. For a more challenging alternative, try a star jump—a much bigger jumping jack with the legs and arms lifting into the air at the same time.

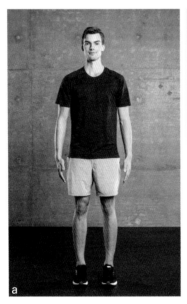 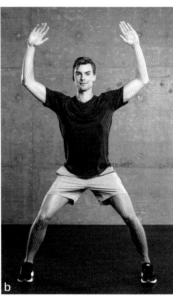

LOW JACK

This exercise begins with the knees slightly bent. Hop the feet out and in repeatedly, staying low and minimizing any vertical displacement. Hands lift only to shoulder height, keeping the elbows bent. As an alternative, try a ground base jumping jack. To begin, start in a straight-arm plank with the hands under the shoulders, the legs extended back and feet positioned slightly wider than hip-width apart, the toes tucked under, and the core engaged. Perform a jumping jack with the feet only: feet together, then jump apart, and back together. As another option, keep the feet tight together and hop both feet to one side and then the other, or kick them up behind into a donkey kick. To increase the challenge, accelerate the tempo of the jumping.

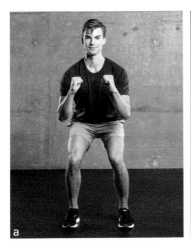 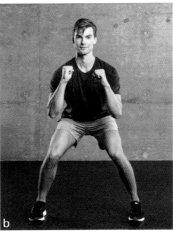

RUNNING ON THE SPOT

Stand with the arms at the sides and start a light jog, alternately swinging the arms in a natural motion. From the jog, begin to lift the knees up higher in front of the body. Increase the pace, driving the knees up and pumping the arms to help create intensity. For a low-impact option, maintain a jog or march.

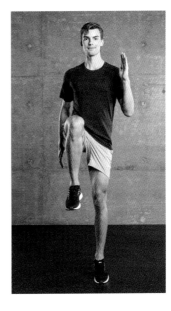

BURPEE

A not-so-favorite favorite! Begin in a standing position with the feet hip-width apart, weight in the heels, and both arms reaching overhead or at the sides. Squat down, placing the hands on the floor in front of you. Shift the weight onto the hands before jumping the legs back into a plank position. Hop the feet back toward the hands and jump up to standing. To increase the challenge, perform a push-up at the bottom of the exercise before hopping the feet toward the hands and jumping up to standing.

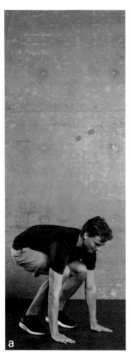 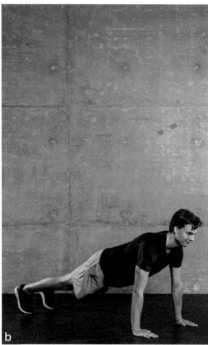 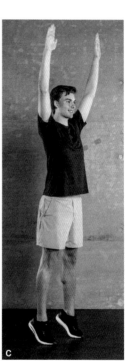

MOUNTAIN CLIMBER

Mountain climbers work the upper body, lower body, and the core. To begin, start in a plank position the hands under the shoulders, the legs extended back and feet positioned slightly wider than hip-width apart, the toes tucked under, and the core engaged. Alternately draw your knees into the chest, switching one leg at a time, using a running-style motion. To increase the challenge, accelerate the pace or draw the knee toward the opposite shoulder.

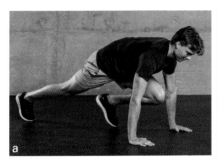 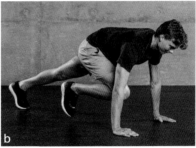

FAST RUN–SQUAT

Alternating fast and low running bursts with a quick drop squat is an effective reactive-style move. Starting in an athletic ready position, stay low and run the feet as fast as possible in place. After about three to five seconds, drop quickly into a squat and hold for two to four seconds. Repeat the pattern, alternating between running and squatting. To make the exercise easier, try a march and drop sequence.

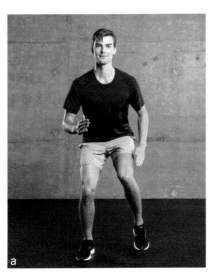 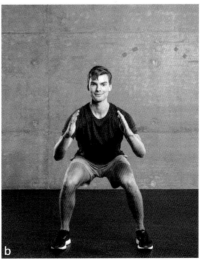

MODERATE

OUT-IN SQUAT WALK

Standing in an athletic ready position, place the hands behind the head, the elbows out to the sides, and the chest lifted. Staying low, step the feet out-out wide, then in-in narrow. Start slowly, and then pick up the pace, keeping the hands on the head, the elbows back, and the lowered hips aligned. Rest and repeat leading with the opposite leg.

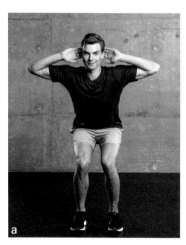 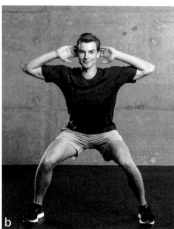

SQUAT, TOUCH, LIFT

EASY

From a standing position, with the feet shoulder-width apart, bend the knees to lower the hips into a squat as you reach the hands down toward the floor. Try to touch or get close to the floor before returning to the start position, lifting the hands to the shoulders or reaching overhead. For additional resistance challenges, hold dumbbells or a small medicine ball, or touch the floor outside of the right foot, center, and then outside of the left foot. Stand, and then repeat, starting to the left.

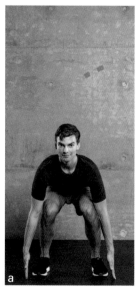 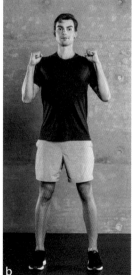

FRONT AND BACK LUNGE

Stand with the feet hip-width apart, the core active, and the arms at the sides. Step forward and bend both knees into a lunge position until the back knee is parallel with the floor. Stand back up, pushing off the front foot, and then taking a step back into a reverse lunge with the same leg. As an option, bring your hands together under the front knee as you lunge forward and reach the arms overhead as you lunge back. Repeat back and forth. To increase the challenge, hold a medicine ball.

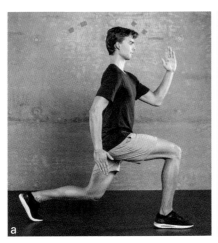 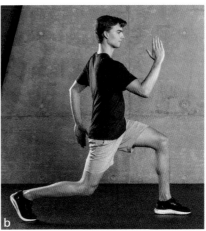

SIDE LUNGE WITH REACH

Stand with the feet hip-width apart and the core engaged. Take a wide step to the right, bending your right knee as you press the hips back. Avoid letting the knee extend past the toe of the bent knee. Push off and return to the start position. Lunge to the opposite side. To increase the challenge, reach down and touch the floor with the outside hand, or hold a medicine ball and touch it to the floor.

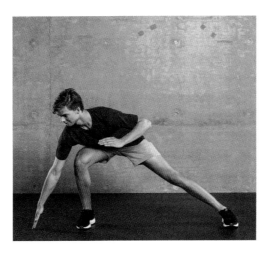

T-BACK PULLS

Begin in a standing position with feet hip-width apart, knees slightly bent, and the arms reaching out to the sides forming a "T." Hinge slightly forward at the hips, engaging through the core. Draw the arms straight back by contracting through the upper back. Pause and return to the starting position and repeat. For variety, include an "I" (arms overhead with thumbs back) and a "Y" (arms overhead and slightly out to the sides) position.

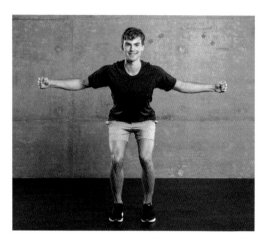

PLANK WITH ARM EXTENDED

Begin in a forearm plank position with the forearms on the floor, elbows under the shoulders, the legs extended back, the feet positioned slightly wider than hip-width apart, and the toes tucked under. Once in alignment, lift into a straight-arm plank and move the right arm out to the side, gently touching the fingertips to the floor. Hold for four to eight seconds. Return to the start position and repeat on the other side. To make the movement easier, stay in a forearm plank position and lower the knees to the floor.

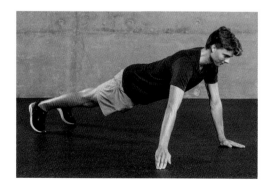

OFFSET PUSH-UP

Begin in a kneeling push-up position. Place one hand lower toward the hip while keeping the other hand under the shoulder. If preferred, increase the challenge and lift up into a fullbody push-up position. Maintain upper body, lower body, and core stability. Perform a push-up for reps, then switch the hands and repeat.

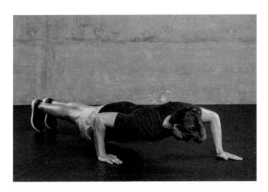

PULL-THROUGH ABS

This is a challenging and unique exercise. In a seated position, extend the legs with the heels on the floor, and the knees slightly bent. Place the hands at the sides, fingertips pointing forward. Lift the glutes up and pull them back between the arms, contracting the core. After pulling the glutes through, push them forward and lift the hips back up. For greater muscle activation, add a triceps dip. Keep the hips up, then bend and straighten the elbows.

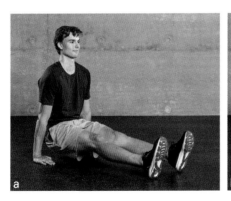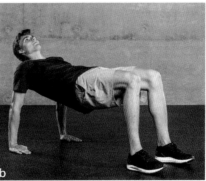

HARD

HARD

HALF-ARC PRESS

Lie faceup on the floor, the arms to the sides with the palms down, the knees slightly bent, and the feet together. Lift the legs off the floor and straight up so the bottoms of the feet face toward the ceiling. Bend the knees and, with control, lower the legs to one side. In an arc fashion, begin by bending the knees in and out pressing the feet up and out following an arc formation from just above the floor on one side, up and over, and all the way to the opposite side. Continue back and forth in both directions.

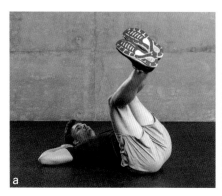
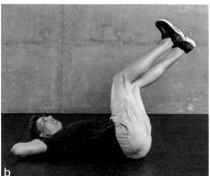

CHAPTER 10

Flexibility Training

Partner stretches are an effective way to round out any workout. As with partner exercises, communication is important so as not to stretch too far, too hard, or too fast. Hold each stretch for approximately 30 to 60 seconds or perform two to four sets of each hold. Avoid holding the breath, and take turns in each of the positions. The following sequence, if followed in order, has a nice flow and covers the major muscle groups.

CHEST STRETCH

Partners stand left shoulder to left shoulder, facing opposite directions. Each partner lifts their left arm, placing it into an L-position. Partners interconnect their top arms, laying one on top of the other, and step forward with the left foot. Open up and feel the stretch in the chest. Repeat on the right side.

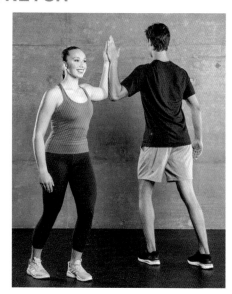

QUADRICEPS STRETCH

Partners stand left shoulder to left shoulder, facing opposite directions, and step an arm's length away from each other out to the side. With the left arms extended, partners grasp each other's left arms just above the shoulder with equal pressure. Next, lift the outside leg, bending the knee and bringing the foot toward the glutes and hold the foot with the opposite hand. Stretch through the front of the leg. Repeat on the other side.

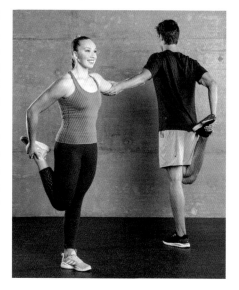

HAMSTRING AND UPPER BACK STRETCH

Partners face each other and interlock forearms, right arms to left arms. As an option, partners can cross the arms. Both partners extend their left legs in front of them, placing the heel on the floor. Shift the weight back, extending through the arms, stretching the upper back, and sinking and lengthening the right leg. Repeat on the left side.

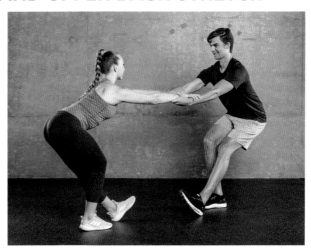

BACK STRETCH

Partners face each other and hold hands with the arms extended, then hinge at the hips and lower the chest toward the floor, moving the feet back as needed. The legs and the arms are straight, gently pulling each other's arms and focusing on the stretch through the back. Next, partners rotate to one side, reaching the arms on that side to the ceiling, feeling the rotation. Hold, then rotate in the opposite direction.

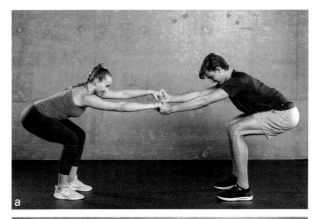

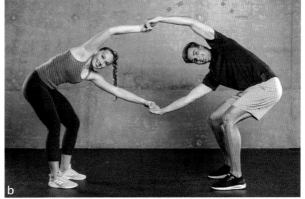

GLUTE STRETCH

Holding onto the partner's forearms, each partner bends the knees slightly and lifts the left leg, placing the left ankle on the right thigh. Use each other for balance while pressing the hips back and deepening the stretch. Repeat on the other side.

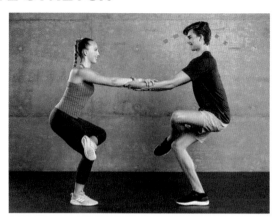

CALF AND HIP FLEXOR STRETCH

Facing each other, press palms to palms with arms at shoulder height, then each partner steps the one foot back approximately one to two feet into an offset stance. While keeping the heel on the floor, lean forward into each other's hands and feel the stretch in the calf and hold. Next, come up onto the toe on the back foot, tuck the hip under, and release the same arm as the back foot, extending back while keeping the opposite hands in contact. Repeat, then switch to the other side.

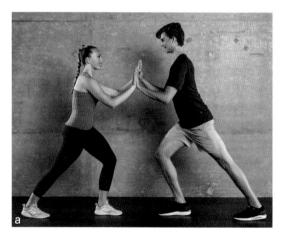

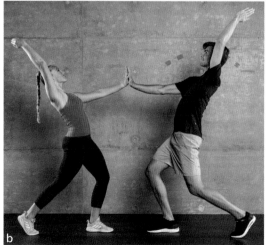

PART III

SAMPLE WORKOUTS

In Part III, you will find a number of different partner workouts to follow. Each workout begins with a brief overview and includes references to the pages where more detailed exercise information can be found. In addition, each workout lists the suggested number of reps or time to completion for each set. Generally, repeating the sets are recommended. Often the first set allows partners to learn the movement pattern and their role in the partner sequence. The subsequent sets strengthen the learning curve and overall experience. The suggested reps and sets are just suggestions and are meant to provide some guidelines. Always work at the intensity that is best for you and your partner. As a basic guideline, if you or your partner fatigues before you complete the suggested reps, the number may be too high and should be adjusted. The same is true if you can easily complete the set. Add more resistance (if applicable) or perform more reps as needed. It is also important to note that some of the workouts may require small equipment. Each workout will list the equipment needed in the overview. Equipment can be substituted, or exercises switched out based on available equipment and space.

As you and your partner try the different workouts and become more familiar with the various combinations, try substituting different exercises. For example, if the workout calls for a squat-based move, try any of the different squatting exercises found throughout the chapters. Experiment and discover new exercises or combinations. Your creativity will keep the workouts fresh and fun!

Before diving into any of the workouts, make sure both you and your partner are warmed up. Chapter 2 reviews the benefits of a proper warm-up. The warm-up doesn't need to be complicated; however, skipping it increases the risk for injury. Note that the warm-up time is not added in the overall workout duration, allowing you to tailor the time to your needs. Finish each workout by stretching, either on your own or with your partner. Lastly, make a plan. Even a little preparation will make the whole experience better. Enjoy!

CHAPTER 11

No-Equipment Workouts

The workouts in this section use the most convenient and easiest equipment to access—your body. These no-equipment workouts range from moderate to more challenging based on the choice of exercises, how each partner is positioned, whether the exercises are done simultaneously or separately, and whether the movements are strength- or cardio-focused.

Double the Fun Workout

This no-equipment workout is an ideal jumping off point for you and your partner to get started. The exercises help partners to get to know each other and include a variety of moves that are meant to create connections. To improve both partners' exercise experience, repeat for a second set. This workout will take 20 minutes to complete.

Double the Fun Workout

Exercise	Photo	Recommended time or reps	Page number
Pushover Press		15-20 seconds	78
Follow the Leader		30 seconds	130
Front Squat Hold		8-12 reps	50

>continued

Double the Fun Workout   >*continued*

Exercise	Photo	Recommended time or reps	Page number
Back-to-Back Walkout		30-60 seconds	77
Plank and Row		8-12 reps	55
Get-Ups		8-12 reps (R and L)	48
Resisted Tabletop		10-15 seconds (R and L)	86
Curl-Up and Jumping Jack		30-60 seconds	145
Rotating Side Planks		6-8 reps	90
Bicycle Crunch		30-60 seconds	69

Together Each Achieves More Workout

The following workout format is challenging because each of the exercises includes working over, on, or against your partner. It also focuses on the lower body and combines cardio and strength exercises. This workout will take approximately 25-30 minutes to complete. For an extra challenge, repeat the entire workout for a second set, with the option to decrease the reps or time if needed.

Together Each Achieves More Workout

Exercise	Photo	Recommended time or reps	Page number
Wide Plank and Agility Footwork		15-30 seconds	136
Pistol Squat		4-6 reps (R and L)	49
Wheelbarrow Push-Up and Squat		8-12 reps	56
Squat and Glute Lift		12-16 reps	51
Donkey Kick		30-60 seconds	138
Glute Bridge Lift		30-60 seconds	83
Down Dog Crawl		45-60 seconds	58
Up-and-Over Abs		60 seconds	72
V-Sit Circle		30 seconds each direction	71

Double Trouble Workout

This full body, no-equipment workout uses your partner as a target (i.e., leaping over your partner's legs) or as part of the exercise (i.e., tabletop and jumping jack). It also includes exercises in which the partner provides additional resistance. If either partner is not comfortable with working on or over each other, separate the moves. For example, in tabletop and jumping jack each partner could simply perform the tabletop and the jumping jack solo, and not on each other as pictured. This workout is more challenging due to the nature of the moves. It is important to include the correct amount of recovery time between sets and it takes approximately 30 minutes to complete.

Double Trouble Workout

Exercise	Photo	Recommended time or reps	Page number
Rotating Squat Jump		30 seconds/side	141
Wall Sit		15-45 seconds	76
Walk Out and Clap		8-12 reps	57
Burpee Jumps		8-12 reps	134

Exercise	Photo	Recommended time or reps	Page number
Tabletop and Jumping Jack		15-30 seconds (R and L)	52
Curl-Up and Give Me 10		30-60 seconds	68
Leg Press		8-12 reps/side	80
Reverse Tabletop and Triceps Dip		30-60 seconds and then switch	53
Resisted Oblique Curl		16-20 reps/side	91

CHAPTER 12

Small-Equipment Workouts

In the following small-equipment workouts, resistance bands and medicine balls are used to add an element of fun and challenge to the exercises. The workouts are strength or cardiofocused, and some include combinations of both. The addition of an athletic-based workout is based on movements that would mimic certain sports or activities. When determining the weight of a medicine ball or the resistance level of a band to use, remember that a chain is only as strong as its weakest link, meaning select the easier equipment choice for the less strong or confident partner.

Let's Band Together Workout

In this cardio- and strength-focused band workout, a minimum of two bands are required depending on the exercises. Some of the cardio-based exercises (i.e., side shuffle) require a bit more space. Also, if the band is placed across the hips, adjust it to a position that is most comfortable and use a light grip to help it stay in place. As noted, if partners possess different fitness levels, choose the correct intensity of resistance bands per individual. A selection of bands might be best. In many of the exercises one partner is doing the reps, while the other partner is holding the band as an anchor. This type of teamwork is beneficial because partners switch roles between working and recovering. The workout will take approximately 30 minutes to complete.

Let's Band Together Workout

Exercise	Photo	Recommended time or reps	Page number
Parachute Band Run		30-45 seconds × 2 sets	110
High Row With Wide Squat		12-16 reps × 2 sets	119
Side Shuffle		30-45 seconds (R and L)	108
Biceps Curl and Side Lunge		8-12 reps (R and L)	117
Front Press and Leap		10-12 (R and L)	111
Boxing Jabs		15-30 seconds × 2 sets	122
Triceps Kickback		12-16 reps × 2 sets	123

Exercise	Photo	Recommended time or reps	Page number
Tap-Down Abs		30-60 seconds × 2 sets	124
Rock and Curl		30-60 seconds × 2 sets	126

Two Be or Not to Be Workout

The following workout intersperses cardio with strength exercises using the resistance band. A minimum of two bands are needed. Some of the exercises, like the chest press, could also be used in small-group training, linking multiple bands together. Other cardio exercises, such as the skier and long jump, are anchored by the partner, and not by linking the bands together. Always make sure the anchor partner maintains good body position and stability. Switch out and use varying band intensities or thicknesses if partners are of different strengths. This workout will take approximately 30 minutes to complete.

Two Be or Not to Be Workout

Exercise	Photo	Recommended time or reps	Page number
Football Run		15-20 seconds × 2 sets	107
Lunge and Rotation		8-12 reps/side	114

>continued

Two Be or Not to Be Workout *>continued*

Exercise	Photo	Recommended time or reps	Page number
Skier		20-30 seconds × 2 sets	106
High Row with Wide Squat		12-16 reps × 2 sets	119
Long Jump		8-10 reps × 2 sets	112
Chest Press		12-16 reps × 2 sets	116
Row and Hop Back		8-10 reps × 2 sets	113
Trunk Rotation		15-30 seconds × 2 sets	120
Oblique Band Curl		16-20 reps (R and L)	127

Pass It On Workout

This medicine ball workout is an appropriate introduction to training with a medicine or plyo ball. Before getting started, try a few light tosses with your partner to ensure the weight is ideal for both of you. When tossing the ball, always make sure your partner is ready and prepared by making eye contact. Switching to a heavier medicine ball for the strength-based exercises is recommended. More space will be required for these throwing-type exercises. This workout focuses on rotational movements and abdominal exercises. It will take approximately 30 minutes to complete.

Pass It On Workout

Exercise	Photo	Recommended time or reps	Page number
Woodchopper		8-12 reps/side	95
Ball Slam		8-12 reps × 2 sets	99
Forward and Backward Lunge and Pass		8-12 reps/side	96
Curl-Up and Pass		30-60 seconds × 2 sets	102

>continued

Pass It On Workout   *>continued*

Exercise	Photo	Recommended time or reps	Page number
Squat to Side Pass		8-12 reps/side	94
Sit and Pass		20-30 seconds × 2 sets	103
Lateral Lunge and Toss		8-12 reps/side	97
Uneven Push-Up and Roll		8-12 reps	100
Seated Pass With Rotation		20-30 seconds/ side × 2 sets	104

Tag, You're It Workout

This full body athletic-focused workout uses the resistance band, medicine ball, and your partner for resistance. The workout begins by elevating the heart rate and then transitions into the strength components. Exercises can be substituted with ones that work similar muscle groups. Choose your favorites or create new renditions of your favorites. The total workout should take approximately 25 minutes to complete.

Tag, You're It Workout

Exercise	Photo	Recommended time or reps	Page number
Resisted Run		15-20 seconds × 2 sets	132
Long Jump and High Jump		30-60 seconds × 2 sets	139
Surfer Pop-Up		4-6 reps × 2 sets	62
Lunge and Rotation		8-12 reps/side	114
Woodchopper		8-12 reps/side	95
Lateral Lunge and Toss		8-12 reps/side	97

>continued

Tag, You're It Workout *>continued*

Exercise	Photo	Recommended time or reps	Page number
Boxing Jabs		15-30 seconds × 2 sets	122
Plank and Row		8-12 reps × 2 sets	55
Oblique Band Curl		16-20 reps/side	127

CHAPTER 13

Cardio and HIIT Workouts

Cardio workouts increase cardiorespiratory response, which cranks up the caloric expenditure and the body's metabolic response both during and after the workout. Using the established training protocols in chapter 8, try the different types of HIIT formats to find some of your favorites. For example, completing one Tabata set takes four minutes. This could be done by choosing one exercise and repeating it, or by alternating between two or four moves. With formats like Tabata, the goal is to shift from work to recovery fairly quickly. Thus, if one of the partner exercises requires more time for set up, it may not work as well; an individual exercise chosen from the solo exercise section in chapter 9 may be preferred. In addition, it would be challenging to perform at maximum effort for this entire workout. Interspersing one or two high-intensity interval sets with lower-intensity cardio is best. Pace yourself based on the exercises themselves. Because these workouts are more challenging, always opt for a low-impact or lower-intensity option if you are just getting started or need to progress a bit slower. Progressing and regressing at the correct rate ensures greater success by feeling more confident that you are doing the movements correctly and at the right intensity.

Teamwork Makes the Dream Work Workout

This all-cardio workout will give each partner a metabolic boost! It is important to note that, although the goal is high intensity, it doesn't have to mean high impact. For example, the football run could be done as a low-impact move, getting lower into a squat and using more upper body movement to increase the intensity. The first four minutes of the workout is a Tabata set, with both partners working and resting at the same time. After recovering for a minimum of two to four minutes, the second part of the workout implements the short-interval hard format, with 30 seconds of work (as intense as possible) followed by 30 seconds of recovery for six sets and six different exercises. Each of the exercise sets allows one partner to be actively working or resting while the other partner is being challenged. The one piece of equipment that is needed in this segment is a resistance band. This is a 12-minute workout.

Teamwork Makes the Dream Work Workout

Exercise	Photo	Recommended time or reps	Page number
Football Run		Tabata: 20 seconds work, 10 seconds recovery × 8 sets	107
1. High-Knees Run		Short intervals hard: 30 seconds work, 30 seconds recovery	131
2. Skier		30 seconds	106
1. Side Shuffle		30 seconds	108
2. Long Jump		30 seconds	112
1. Parachute Band Run		30 seconds	110
2. Plank Leap		30 seconds	137

Twice Bitten, Once Shy Workout

This HIIT workout is a 20-minute double-set cardio blast focusing on short-interval sets and is not recommended for beginners unless they have a good cardio base and a strong core and upper body. As one partner is working hard, the other partner is also involved in the exercise sequence, such as holding a plank. The format of work to active recovery allows for 15 to 30 seconds of work followed by a recovery time that is dependent on the difficulty of the exercises. Repeat for two to four sets, starting from the beginning of the workout. With many non-cardio positions on the hands, be aware of the correct wrist position and modify as necessary.

Twice Bitten, Once Shy Workout

Exercise	Photo	Recommended time or reps	Page number
Walkout Ankle Taps		15-30 seconds	142
Down Dog Crawl		15-30 seconds	58
Wide Plank and Agility Footwork		15-30 seconds	136
Burpee Jumps		15-30 seconds	134
Tabletop and Jumping Jack		15-30 seconds/ side	52

>continued

Twice Bitten, Once Shy Workout   *>continued*

Exercise	Photo	Recommended time or reps	Page number
Donkey Kick		15-30 seconds	138
Narrow Push-Up and Hop Over		15-30 seconds	144
Curl-Up and Jumping Jack		15-30 seconds	145

CHAPTER 14

Full Body Workouts

Variety certainly is the spice of life when it applies to exercise programs. The more interesting the workout, the more enjoyable training tends to be, and if you add a partner, you double the fun. There are infinite ways to put together workouts. Stacked and supersetting workouts can include exercises that can be complementary or opposing, or follow certain patterns. Tri-setting includes three different or complementary exercises back-to-back with no rest in between. Superslow training involves lifting and lowering at a very slow pace. Once you have mastered a format, mix it up and try new ones to avoid exercise plateaus or boredom.

Stack Attack Workout

This full body workout stacks three exercises. Each set begins with a cardio exercise, transitions to a lower body–focused exercise, and finishes with an upper body–focused exercise. Repeat each segment in order twice before moving on to the next three exercises. To increase the challenge, eliminate the recovery in between segments to be more tri-set focused. For a less challenging workout, eliminate the cardio segment and replace with an abdominal or core-focused exercise—try the back extension, straight-leg lift or curl-up and give me 10. The total workout should take approximately 30 minutes to complete.

Stack Attack Workout

Exercise	Photo	Recommended time or reps	Page number
1. Squat Jump to High 10		30 seconds	140

>continued

Stack Attack Workout >continued

Exercise	Photo	Recommended time or reps	Page number
2. Pistol Squat		4-6 reps (R and L)	49
3. Kneeling Push-Up With Rotation		8-10 reps (R and L)	63
1. Rotating Squat Jump		30 seconds/side	141
2. Wall Sit		15-45 seconds	76
3. Snowboarder		30 seconds/side	61
1. Long Jump and High Jump		30-60 seconds	139

Exercise	Photo	Recommended time or reps	Page number
2. Squat and Glute Lift		12-15 reps	51
3. Handstand		2-6 sets	66

What's Not to Resist? Workout

The following exercise sequence requires no equipment and focuses entirely on partner-resisted exercises. Each partner takes an active role in the workout either by performing the exercise or providing the resistance in the exercise. Good communication is required to determine the amount of pressure to be applied. The total workout should take approximately 15-20 minutes to complete one set.

What's Not to Resist? Workout

Exercise	Photo	Recommended time or reps	Page number
Lunge and Press		30 seconds/side	79
Back-to-Back Walkout		30-60 seconds	77

>continued

What's Not to Resist? Workout >*continued*

Exercise	Photo	Recommended time or reps	Page number
Pushover Press		15-20 seconds	78
Resisted Front and Side Raise		6-8 reps/ position	85
Leg Press		8-12 reps (R and L)	80
Side Plank Hold		8-12 reps/side	88
Glute Bridge Bicycle		30-60 seconds	84
Resisted Hamstring Curl		8-12 reps/side	82
Resisted Push-Up		8-12 reps	87

CHAPTER 15

Specialty Workouts

The following three workouts have specific themes. The first sequence focuses on the abs and core—two often-requested areas to exercise. It is important to note that, although the focus is on the torso, there is no such thing as spot reducing. You could perform hundreds of abdominal exercises and never lose body fat if that is all you do. A well-rounded program for fat loss includes cardio and strength training, lifestyle changes, and healthy, nutrition-based eating. If you like, create your own workouts that focus on a specific area to train. For example, choose 8 to 10 exercises for the lower body or upper body. The second workout is fun and kid friendly, and takes into account different body sizes. Using some small pieces of equipment (bands and balls) makes the workout more interesting. The final workout in this section includes solo exercises. Neither partner is using equipment nor in contact with each other. Rather, they are working beside each other and alternating between different exercises.

Ab-Fusion Not Confusion Workout

Even though there is no such thing as spot reducing, focusing on one area of the body can be an optional way to train. It provides opportunities to thoroughly fatigue the muscles, or to highlight stronger or weaker areas within the muscular unit. In the following workout, the abs are the star of the show, and the core is activated throughout. The workout can be performed with a plyo ball and band or without equipment by substituting core favorites like the half-arc press, pull-through abs, or plank with arm extended found in chapter 9. Be sure to warm up first and use a mat for greater comfort. The total workout should take approximately 20-25 minutes to complete.

Ab-Fusion Not Confusion Workout

Exercise	Photo	Recommended time or reps	Page number
Walk Out and Clap		30 seconds × 1-2 sets	57
Straight-Leg Lift		8-12 reps × 2 sets	67
Curl-Up and Give Me 10		30-60 seconds × 2 sets	68
Resisted Tabletop		10-15 seconds/ side × 2 sets	86
Up-and-Over Abs		60 seconds × 1-2 sets	72

Exercise	Photo	Recommended time or reps	Page number
Rotating Side Planks		6-8 reps × 1-2 sets	90
Tap-Down Abs		30 seconds × 2 sets	124
V-Sit Circle		15 seconds/ direction	71
Bicycle Crunch		30-60 seconds × 2 sets	69
Seated Pass With Rotation		20-30 seconds/ side	104
Back Extension		30-45 seconds × 2 sets	73

Dueling Dynamos Workout

This is a fun workout to try with a younger family member or friend. It is designed with an adult and child pairing in mind, but with some experience and supervision, younger kids or siblings could partner up and work out with each other. This workout uses a variety of equipment (resistance band, medicine ball, and body weight) and focuses on keeping the exercises interesting, fun, and kid friendly. The workout is quick and should take approximately 20 minutes. Crank up the tunes (kid approved) and let the fun begin.

Dueling Dynamos Workout

Exercise	Photo	Recommended time or reps	Page number
Follow the Leader		15-20 seconds × 2 sets	130
Front Squat Hold		6-8 reps	50
Lunge and Press		6-8 reps per side	79
Squat to Side Pass		6-8 reps per side	94
Row and Hop Back		8-10 reps	113

Exercise	Photo	Recommended time or reps	Page number
Ball Slam		6-8 reps × 2 sets	99
Front Press and Leap		6-8 reps per side	111
Leapfrog		20-30 seconds × 2 sets	133
Crab and Reach		6-8 reps per side	60
Plank Leap		10-15 seconds × 2 sets	137
Curl-Up and Pass		15-20 seconds × 2 sets	102

Tandem Tune-Up Workout

This partner solo workout is all about being together, but apart. In this workout each partner performs an exercise separate from their partner, and then swaps moves. For example, partner A performs the burpee and partner B performs the T-back pulls. Once the sets are completed, partner A does the T-back pulls and partner B performs the burpee. Each exercise is completed in approximately 15 to 30 seconds, increasing over time to 45 to 60 seconds. Timing the sets will be easier to manage versus trying to count reps. Include 10 to 15 seconds of recovery between sets, or longer if needed. Each exercise pairing includes a cardio and strength focus. Repeat the sequence twice to ensure the exercises are completed on both the right and left sides. Complete the workout, finishing with the three core-focused exercises at the end. The workout should take approximately 30 minutes to complete.

Tandem Tune-Up Workout

Exercise	Photo	Recommended time or reps	Page number
1. Jumping Jack		15-30 seconds	148
2. Front and Back Lunge		15-30 seconds	153
1. Running on the Spot		15-30 seconds	149
2. Out–In Squat Walk		15-30 seconds	152

Exercise	Photo	Recommended time or reps	Page number
1. Fast Run–Squat		15-30 seconds	151
2. Side Lunge With Reach		15-30 seconds	153
1. Burpee		15-30 seconds	150
2. T-Back Pulls		15-30 seconds	154
1. Low Jack		15-30 seconds	149
2. Offset Push-Up		15-30 seconds	155
1. Mountain Climber		15-30 seconds	151
2. Squat, Touch, Lift		15-30 seconds	152

>continued

Tandem Tune-Up Workout   *>continued*

Exercise	Photo	Recommended time or reps	Page number
1. Pull-Through Abs		15-30 seconds	155
2. Plank With Arm Extended		15-30 seconds	154
3. Half-Arc Press		15-30 seconds	156

CHAPTER 16

Flexibility Training Workout

Dessert following dinner is a lovely way to finish a meal. Unlike dessert that is not always good for you, flexibility training is not only beneficial, but recommended after every workout.

Chapter 10 reviews the numerous benefits of flexibility training and the correct technique. Partner stretching includes both static and passive stretches. A passive stretch allows you to relax while your partner intensifies the stretch by adding some external pressure, for example, pulling you a little deeper into the hamstring and upper back stretch. A static stretch involves holding a stretch for a period of time without movement.

Stretching Along and Not Alone Workout

The following stretches are done together and in contact with your partner. The sequence flows from start to finish and includes stretches for the major muscle groups in the lower body and the upper body. Hold each stretch for a minimum of 30 seconds or longer if time permits, and repeat if possible. The total stretch sequence should take approximately 8-10 minutes to complete. As in the other partner exercises, communication is important. Pulling too hard or putting too much pressure on your partner in a stretch can cause them to extend farther than intended. Ensure that you are breathing in a way that complements the stretches. Inhale to prepare to move and exhale as you both hold the stretches.

Table 16.1 Stretching Along and Not Alone Workout

Exercise	Photo	Recommended time or reps	Page number
Chest Stretch		30-60+ seconds	158
Quadriceps Stretch		30-60+ seconds	158
Hamstring and Upper Back Stretch		30-60+ seconds	159
Back Stretch		30-60+ seconds	159
Glute Stretch		30-60+ seconds	160
Calf and Hip Flexor Stretch		30-60+ seconds	160

APPENDIX A

Personal Training for Partner Workouts

Partner training is an excellent way for a personal trainer to increase training revenue. With limited time available each day and within the week, doubling up on your client base both hourly and weekly has a financial payoff. More revenue per hour (charging two clients versus one) is a better financial use of your time. In addition, clients get better results when they exercise more often. Perhaps a client can't afford weekly one-on-one sessions, but they may be able to afford partner workouts. Encouraging partner workouts also broadens a trainer's repertoire of exercise options and helps create interactive and engaging sessions. This can result in a more motivating training environment. Partners also tend to work harder when there is a little bit of competition thrown into the mix. Lastly, less equipment is needed (or none at all) for partner workouts, and a trainer can train clients across a wide range of venues, from studios to homes.

Successful Partner Workout Implementation Tips for Personal Trainers

After considering which clients would benefit from partner training and prior to delving into your first session, set aside some time to plan and prepare the workout. Training sessions that are most successful are the ones that are most carefully mapped out.

- *Planning.* Take time to plan the workout. Each partner session should include decisions on exercise choice, frequency, intensity, time, repetitions, rest, and sets. Make sure there is a balance and flow between target muscles, foundational movements, positioning, and equipment.

- *Practice.* Before any session, test each exercise with a partner so you are aware of how the movements feel and are conscious of any positioning complexities and how to progress or regress the movements.

- *Communication.* Make sure your cues (directions) are clear and concise. Be prepared to use different cuing techniques to explain the same movement. Good communication has content—the message, motivation—a stimulus, and emotion—the responsive feelings to the message.

- *Demo.* Demonstrating an exercise is an efficient teaching technique. Good communication uses both visual and verbal messaging. Most information processing is visual so observing the partner exercise is important.

- *Focus.* Ensure both partners are focused and present during the exercises. Even the partner who is the anchor still needs to be engaged in the process. Balance the exercises between both partners being active and being the anchor or recovering. Encourage both partners to maintain concentration and work intensity.

- *Safety.* Not all exercises are suited for all partners. Be ready to pivot and change. Regressing an exercise doesn't necessarily equate to an easier move. Ask yourself if this is the correct exercise or movement to meet the needs of the client and to be successful.

- *Encouragement.* Being an engaging and positive trainer is the best way to create adoring training fans. Bring out the best in your clients by providing technique reminders and specific and positive feedback.

Successful Partner Training in Group Settings

Many fitness professionals have multiple roles within the fitness industry. Because of this diversity, these functions can encompass teaching group classes, training one-on-one, coaching, and even program directing at a club or studio level. When teaching fitness classes or leading group training, partner drills are an excellent way to add variety to a workout and help members connect. Group participants often see each other regularly in the workout environment, but they don't always interact or engage. Partner drills can change that. However, there is still a level of discomfort that is associated with having to partner with a stranger. It is the trainer's role to mitigate those feelings through some simple housekeeping tips.

First, avoid planning the entire group workout around partner exercises. The goal is to have a bit of fun by adding a few exercises into the mix here and there. For greater success, plan for a maximum of two to four partner exercises. In addition, choose exercises that use a piece of equipment as a buffer versus touching hands. Introduce the partner drills during the second half of the workout instead of right at the start. The feel-good workout response will ideally help participants be more willing to trying something new. You may also want to alternate a partner exercise with an individual exercise such as a balance or agility move.

To get started, ask members to find a partner. If there is an odd number that is not a problem; simply create a group of three. Position the partners so that everyone is facing the same direction and spaced out evenly. Ideally, you would encourage people to find a partner who is similar in strength, height, and ability, but that is not always possible. Start with a basic exercise (e.g., high row with wide squat in chapter 7) that will work well with partners who may have different fitness abilities. Keep the bands anchored in one spot versus complicated anchor positions. Looping them once works well. To start, partner A does a high row, repeated by partner B. In this example, alternating the move allows partners to work at their own level. Next, transition the move to simultaneously rowing.

Lastly, add more challenge by increasing the resistance (e.g., stepping farther away from the anchor point in the center) or add complexity by including movement (e.g., wide squats). Repeating the same exercise with a slight variation allows for a successful learning curve and the integration of more movement. In this example, adding any type of a lower body move to the row adds variety and challenge. Be sure to cue technique tips and decide whether to use a time- or a rep-based format for keeping track of the sets.

Successful Partner Workout Cueing Tips for Personal Trainers

As a personal trainer, leading partner training sessions or small groups requires a slightly different approach than training one-on-one. Being able to communicate well is a dynamic process and allows clients to process information correctly.

When working simultaneously with two clients, chances are each client may hear or interpret the same cue differently, or the cue may resonate with one more than the other. Having different prompts helps clients process information effectively.

Here are some examples of different cueing techniques to get your message across clearly.

- *Anatomical cues.* Describe the body part and its associated action: Contract and tighten the quadriceps muscles.
- *Kinesthetic cues.* Describe how the action would feel and the awareness and positioning of the muscles and body: Imagine holding a pencil between your shoulder blades.
- *Explanatory cues.* Clarify the purpose of the exercise or drill: The goal is to focus on the legs moving in a circular fashion.
- *Adjustment cues.* Provide movement corrections: Avoid letting the knee move past the front toe.
- *Motivational cues.* Be enthusiastic and inspiring: You've got this, you can do it! Only 15 seconds to go!
- *Complimentary cues.* Offer encouragement and positive feedback: You did such a great job keeping up the intensity for the entire set!

Lastly, try to balance task cues with reflective questions. A task cue is a directive telling the client what to do, for example, "Keep the spine long." A reflective cue provokes an internal response from the listener. For example, instead of saying, "Keep the spine long," a reflective question would be, "Can you feel your spine lengthen?" The listener would internally evaluate if their spine was lengthening, and if the answer was no, they know what should be happening and can respond. After the question is asked, provide an option to apply the information, for example, "Can you lengthen your spine for the next 30 seconds as you hold the plank?"

Because all parts of a workout require different types of cueing, make sure to mix it up. Practice helps; cueing well is not always as easy as it seems. Take the time to try different techniques and learn how to better communicate in both partner or group training situations.

Successful Partner Workout Training With Sport Teams

Introducing athletes to partner workouts has incredible benefits outside of the physical training. First and foremost, teammates must trust each other. Partner workouts build trust. As a kid, you may have played the trust game. You would stand with your friend behind you, facing the same direction. If you were in front, you would keep your body completely straight and then let yourself fall directly back toward the floor. But before you would come crashing down, your buddy would catch you before you hit the floor. You blindly trusted that your friend would not let you get hurt. This example, like some of the exercises in the book, requires trust in your partner.

If your partner is jumping over your back in the leapfrog exercise, you have to feel confident that your partner is not going to step on your foot or press too hard on your back. If you are the quarterback on the football team, you have to trust that your defense is going to protect you. Trust encompasses many sports.

The other benefit of implementing partner workouts with sports teams is communication. Whether you are on a court, rink, or field, you have to talk to your teammates to let them know where you are or what your opponents are doing. In many of the exercises, partners must communicate with each other regarding positioning, how much resistance is needed, and even how much time or how many reps are left in a set before switching roles. Young athletes are particularly shy at communicating. Doing drills that help break the ice and build comfort with teammates is invaluable.

Lastly are the physical and mental benefits of partner workouts. Many of the exercises are really fun and a little daring, which keeps athletes' interest high. It also seems less like exercise and more like play when you are doing fun moves. Crawling underneath a teammate in the down dog crawl set (see chapter 5), jumping over them in the plank leap (see chapter 8), or taking out some aggression in the ball slam (see chapter 7) are challenging and effective activities.

Most of the exercises in partner workouts cross over well to all sports. Whether you implement a few in a warm-up or design an entire training session, partner exercises will capture the players' interest and provide benefits both on and off the court.

Successful Virtual Partner Training

For trainers taking a more proactive approach and using virtual training as a part of their business, it would be beneficial to invest in a proper camera and microphone system for video production. When filming, make sure the space is well lit, and avoid any background light. For example, if there is a window in the space, position yourself so that it isn't behind you. Rather, the light should be directly on your face and body; natural light is always best. Lighting from above can cast shadows and is not the most flattering.

If you are a trainer planning to charge for any type of training session, the experience should be of a higher quality than friends just deciding to exercise together over any virtual platform. Create a professional environment with proper sound and lighting for a quality virtual session, and chances are it will be a win-win for everyone.

If you are providing personal training online, make sure you have done your homework and purchased the correct liability insurance to train virtually. One of the caveats for many coverage choices is the ability to see your clients and for them to see you.

Managing and Charging for Partner Training Sessions

Establishing an income-based personal training business means being resourceful with how you schedule and manage your time. With only so many working hours in a week, and a fairly physical job, blocking your time with one-on-one clients only is not ideal, nor is it financially prudent. If you train Jane for one hour at 60 dollars or you partner train Jane and her friend Sarah for 90 dollars, not only is the session less expensive for Jane, 45 dollars versus 60 dollars, but you earn more money per hour. Partner or small-group training fills that same one-hour spot, but at a much higher revenue share. Thus, it is more beneficial to add more partner training to your business. Find out what others in your training area are charging; this is dependent on the area of the world in which you live and work. Check out the studios or research online. Individual partner training fees are commonly less than what a client would pay for a one-on-one session. Commonly, the hourly partner fee is 50 percent more. For example, if you normally charge 60 dollars for an individual session, you'd charge 90 dollars for a partner training session.

To make your training packages more appealing and marketable, consider offering value-added services like complementary couple vacation training plans, package transfers, a virtual session, or bring-a-friend-for-free perks.

Today's customers are accustomed to quick and easy service, regardless of their age or demographic. Make communication, scheduling, and payment options as easy as possible by using an online platform. If you combine these details with a fantastic partner training session, your business will be booming.

APPENDIX B

SWEAT Self-Worksheet

Use the following worksheet to reflect on your exercise successes, to list any obstacles to your success (either in the past or in the future), and to highlight what you truly want to achieve on your fitness journey (refer to chapter 4). This sheet can be filled out alone or together with your partner. Completing it with your partner is a great way to share previous struggles and to solidify your goals by creating accountability checks. By being aware of each other's goals and challenges, you can better help and support each other in the process.

Date: _____ Name: _____

Next reflection date: _____ (in 3 months)

Strengths, Weaknesses, Excuses, Aspirations, Targets

Reflect and respond with three to five answers to the following questions:

1. **Strengths.** List your strengths as they relate to your current health and fitness or your fitness journey to date.

   _____
   _____
   _____
   _____
   _____
   _____

2. **Weaknesses.** List your weaknesses as they relate to your health and fitness goals or to challenges you have faced.

   _____
   _____
   _____
   _____
   _____
   _____

3. **Excuses.** List your favorite or most often used excuses or obstacles for not working out or not achieving your goals.

_____

_____

_____

_____

_____

_____

4. **Aspirations.** What would you like to achieve? Your aspirations could include something as simple as how you want to feel, or they could involve multifaceted goals and achievements.

_____

_____

_____

_____

_____

_____

5. **Targets.** Your targets are your goals. These should include both small and large goals, and your goal-achievement date. The more specific and realistic you can be, the better.

_____

_____

_____

_____

_____

_____

WORKS CITED

CHAPTER 1

Bergland, C. 2016. "Having Social Bonds is the No. 1 Way to Optimize Your Health." *The Athlete's Way* (blog), *Psychology Today*. January 14, 2016. www.psychologytoday.com/ca/blog/the-athletes-way/201601/having-social-bonds-is-the-no-1-way-optimize-your-health.

Boldt, A. 2018. "The Difference Between Muscular Strength & Muscular Endurance." Last modified January 30, 2018. www.livestrong.com/article/154326-the-difference-between-muscular-strength-muscular-endurance/.

Daussin, F.N., J. Zoll, S.P. Dufour, E. Ponsot, E. Lonsdorfer-Wolf, S. Doutreleau, B. Mettauer, F. Piquard, B. Geny, and R. Richard. 2008. "Effect of Interval Versus Continuous Training on Cardiorespiratory and Mitochondrial Functions: Relationship to Aerobic Performance Improvements in Sedentary Subjects." *American Journal of Physiology. Regulatory, Integrative, and Comparative Physiology* 295 (1): R264-72. doi: 10.1152/ajpregu.00875.2007.

Kravitz, L. 2006. "A NEAT New Strategy for Weight Control." *IDEA Fitness Journal* 3 (4), 24-25. www.unm.edu/~lkravitz/Article%20folder/NeatLK.html.

Kravitz, L. 2014. "ACSM Information on High-Intensity Interval Training." www.acsm.org/docs/default-source/files-for-resource-library/high-intensity-interval-training.pdf?sfvrsn=b0f72be6_2.

McCall, P. 2019. *Smarter Workouts*: *The Science of Exercise Made Simple*. Champaign, IL: Human Kinetics.

Magal, M. and M. Scheinowitz. 2018. "Benefits and Risks Associated with Physical Activity." In *ACSM's Guidelines for Exercise Testing and Prescription*, 10th edition, edited by American College of Sports Medicine, 1-21. Philadelphia: Wolters Kluwer. www.acsm.org/docs/default-source/publications-files/acsm-guidelines-download-10th-edabf32a97415a400e9b3be594a6cd7fbf.pdf?sfvrsn=aaa6d2b2_0.

Magness, S. 2016. "A Brief History of Interval Training: The 1800's to Now." Last modified August 18, 2016. www.scienceofrunning.com/2016/08/a-brief-history-of-interval-training-the-1800s-to-now.html?v=47e5dceea252.

Potteiger, J. 2018. "Exercise Science: A Systems Approach." In *ACSM's Introduction to Exercise Science*, 3rd edition, 57-100. Philadelphia: Wolters Kluwer Health. www.acsm.org/docs/default-source/publications-files/intro-to-exsci-3_sample-chapter-3.pdf?sfvrsn=2c9320fb_8.

Riebe, D., B.A. Franklin, P.D. Thompson, C.E. Garber, G.P. Whitfield, M. Magal, and L.S. Pescatello. 2015. "Updating ACSM's Recommendations for Exercise Preparticipation Health Screening." *Medicine & Science in Sports & Exercise* 47 (8): 2473-2479. www.acsm.org/docs/default-source/files-for-resource-library/updating_acsm_s_recommendations_for_exercise-28-(1).pdf?sfvrsn=3aa47c01_4.

Setton, M., P. Desan, D. Park, M. Toribio-Mateas, T. Arciero, S. Qureshi. n.d. "Relationships and Happiness." Accessed April 22, 2021. www.pursuit-of-happiness.org/science-of-happiness/relationships_and_happiness/.

Thompson, D.L. 2008. "Fitness Focus Copy-and-Share: Flexibility." *ACSM's Health & Fitness Journal* 12 (5): 5. doi: 10.1249/FIT.0b013e318184516b.

Valdivia, O.D., M.A. Martin Cañada, F.Z. Ortega, J.J. Antequera Rodríguez, M. Fernández Sánchez. 2009. "Changes in Flexibility According to Gender and Educational Stage." *Apunts. Medicina de l'Esport,* 44 (161): 10-17. www.apunts.org/en-changes-in-flexibility-according-gender-articulo-13135385.

Zuhl, M. and L. Kravitz. 2012. "HIIT vs Continuous Endurance Training: Battle of the Aerobic Titans." *IDEA Fitness Journal,* 9 (2), 34-40. www.unm.edu/~lkravitz/Article%20folder/HIITvsCardio.html.

CHAPTER 2

Can-Fit-Pro Fitness Instructor Specialist. 2009-2010. *The Essential Resource for the Can-Fit-Pro Fitness Instructor Specialist Certification*. Page 4.

Dintiman, G. and B. Ward. 2003. *Sports Speed*. 3rd ed. Champaign, IL: Human Kinetics.

Langton, B. and J. King. 2018. "Utilizing Body Weight Training With Your Personal Training Clients." *ACSM s Health & Fitness Journal* 22 (6): 44-51. doi: 10.1249/FIT.0000000000000433.

Magal. M. and M. Scheinowitz. 2018. "Benefits and Risks Associated with Physical Activity." In *ACSM's Guidelines for Exercise Testing and Prescription,* 10th edition, edited by American College of Sports Medicine, 1-21. Philadelphia: Wolters Kluwer. www.acsm.org/docs/default-source/publications-files/acsm-guidelines-download-10th-edabf32a97415a400e9b3be594a6cd7fbf.pdf?sfvrsn=aaa6d2b2_0.

McCall, P. 2019. *Smarter Workouts*: *The Science of Exercise Made Simple.* Champaign, IL: Human Kinetics.

CHAPTER 3

Australian Fitness Academy. 2019. "Upper Body Plyometric Exercises." *Australian Fitness Academy* (blog), *Australian Fitness Academy.* October 25, 2019. www.fitnesseducation.edu.au/blog/fitness/upper-body-plyometric-exercises/.

Chu, D. and G. Myer. 2013. *Plyometrics*. Champaign, IL: Human Kinetics.

Elite Performance Institute. n.d.. "Variable Resistance Training (VRT) – Bands & Chains." (blog), *Elite Performance Institute*. January 5, 2020. www.epicertification.com/variable-resistance-training-vrt-bands-chains/.

Freytag, C. 2020. "Benefits of Resistance Bands for Strength Training." Last modified October 21, 2020. www.verywellfit.com/resistance-bands-strength-training-3498170.

Harvard Medical School. 2019. "Join the Resistance: Resistance Bands Offer an Easy Way to Get an All-Around Strength Workout at Home." Last modified August 2019. www.health.harvard.edu/staying-healthy/join-the-resistance.

Heffernan, C. 2020. "The Long History of the Medicine Ball." Last modified January 29, 2020. https://physicalculturestudy.com/2020/01/29/the-long-history-of-the-medicine-ball/.

Hodanbosi, C. 1996. "The First and Second Laws of Motion." Last modified August 1996. www.grc.nasa.gov/www/k-12/WindTunnel/Activities/first2nd_lawsf_motion.html.

Iversen, V.M., P.J. Mork, O. Vasseljen, R. Bergquist, and M.S. Fimland. 2017. "Multiple-Joint Exercises Using Elastic Resistance Bands vs. Conventional Resistance-Training Equipment: A Cross-Over Study." *European Journal of Sport Science* 17 (8): 973-982.

Page, P. and T. Ellenbecker. 2020. *Strength Band Training.* 3rd ed. Champaign: IL: Human Kinetics.

Payne, A. 2019. "Sagittal, Frontal and Transverse Plane: Movements and Exercises." *NASM Workout Plans* (blog), *National Academy of Sports Medicine.* June 4, 2019. https://blog.nasm.org/exercise-programming/sagittal-frontal-traverse-planes-explained-with-exercises.

Raineri, M. 2015."EMG Studies Show Best Exercises!" Last modified September 21, 2015. www.bodybuilding.com/fun/teen-mark4.htm.

Silva Lopes, J.S., A.F. Machado, J.K. Micheletti, A. Castilho de Almeida, A.P. Cavina, and C.M. Pastre. 2019. "Effects of Training with Elastic Resistance Versus Conventional Resistance on Muscular Strength: A Systematic Review and Metaanalysis." *Sage Open Medicine* 7: 1-7. www.ncbi.nlm.nih.gov/pmc/articles/PMC6383082/.

Stoppani, J. 2020. "The Science of Strength Bands." Last modified July 28, 2020. www.jimstoppani.com/training/science-of-strength-bands.

Walker, O. 2016. "Elastic-Resistance Training." Last modified June 19, 2016. www.scienceforsport.com/elastic-resistance-training/.

CHAPTER 4

Deschenes, M.R. and C.E. Garber. 2018. "General Principles of Exercise Prescription." In *ACSM's Guidelines for Exercise Testing and Prescription*, 10th ed., edited by American College of Sports Medicine, 126-129. Philadelphia: Wolters Kluwer. www.acsm.org/docs/default-source/publications-files/acsms-exercise-testing-prescription.pdf?sfvrsn=111e9306_4

DeSimone, G. 2019. "The Tortoise Factor—Get FITT." *ACSM's Health & Fitness Journal* 23 (2): 3-4. doi: 10.1249/FIT.0000000000000456.

Doran, G.T. 1981. "There's a S.M.A.R.T. Way to Write Management's Goals and Objectives." *Management Review* 70 (11): 35-36.

U.S. Department of Health and Human Services. 2018. *Physical Activity Guidelines for Americans*, 2nd ed. Washington, D.C.: U.S. Department of Health and Human Services.

ABOUT THE AUTHOR

Krista Popowych, BHKin, is a renowned presenter and instructor of group fitness, personal training, and fitness management. She has traveled extensively to share her passion for fitness by educating instructors and trainers at conferences and speaking engagements across the globe. She received the prestigious international IDEA Fitness Instructor of the Year award and has also been recognized for her countless contributions to the continual education of fitness professionals across Canada, receiving canfitpro's Canadian Presenter of the Year honor three times.

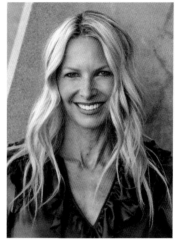

Popowych's career has spanned the many transformations and innovations that have taken the fitness industry to where it is today. In addition to a degree in human kinetics (kinesiology), focusing on instructing and coaching, she holds specialty certifications as a Keiser indoor cycling master trainer and a Balanced Body integrated movement specialist, and she has multiple training certifications in disciplines such as Pilates, yoga, stability ball, TRX suspension training, kickboxing, BOSU, fitness trampoline, and Barre. She also holds leadership certifications from canfitpro as a Fitness Instructor Specialist (FIS) and a Personal Trainer Specialist (PTS), and she is a certified BCRPA Trainer of Fitness Leaders (TFL). She is the global director of group education for Keiser and the cocreator of The Ride, an on-demand indoor cycling and fitness platform.

As a dynamic on-camera fitness instructor, Popowych has hosted and cohosted one of Canada's most widely televised health and fitness shows and has hundreds of hours of featured video fitness and education content. In addition to being a freelance writer with contributions to *IDEA Fitness Journal*, *American Fitness*, *Australian Fitness Network*, *Club Industry Fitness Business Pro*, and *canfitpro Magazine*, she has been a fitness columnist and a source expert in magazines such as *Shape* and *Chatelaine*. Krista also gives back to the community by mentoring university kinesiology students and supporting various fundraising initiatives, sharing her time and talents. She is a board member and consultant for numerous influential fitness companies, contributing her insights and real-world advice. Krista lives in Vancouver, Canada, with her husband, son, and daughter. She loves spending time with all of her family and friends, keeping active, having fun, always learning, and living each day with a grateful heart.

You read the book—now complete the companion CE exam to earn continuing education credit!

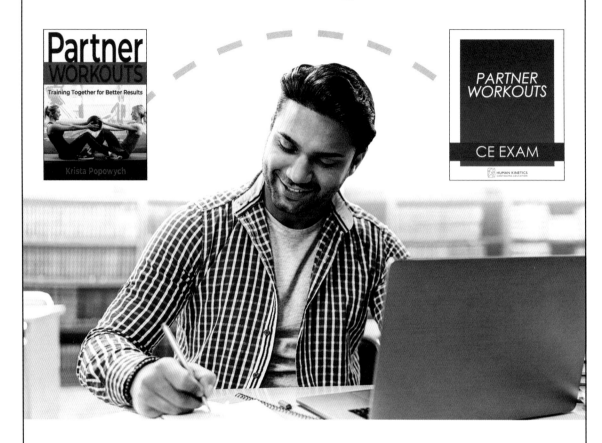

Find and purchase the companion CE exam here:
US.HumanKinetics.com/collections/CE-Exam
Canada.HumanKinetics.com/collections/CE-Exam

50% off the companion CE exam with this code

PW2022

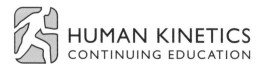